WATER FASTING

Autophagy, Weight Loss, Anti-aging, and Healing Your Own Body Fast for Beginners

DANA WELLS

Water is the driving force of all nature.

Leonardo da Vinci

WATER FASTING

Autophagy, Weight Loss, Anti-aging, and Healing
Your Own Body Fast for Beginners

DANA WELLS

Contents

any medical condition, they should seek immediate medical attention and not use this book in place of actual medical expertise. Readers should never delay medical and healthcare treatment, ignore previous advice and diagnosis, or halt their current medical treatment because of the information in this book. The author of this book is not a healthcare professional and has no prior medical experience in relation to the included subjects. The reader holds sole responsibility for their own personal actions and negligence in regard to the contents of this book. The author does not hold any legal or personal responsibility for any injury, misinterpretation, fraudulent behavior, negligence, or death that may result from this book. All content and advice should be read and practiced with care and consideration when participating in the mentioned activities. Common sense should be used by the participating party in order to receive the best and safest results.

Introduction

Congratulations on downloading *Water Fasting: Autophagy, Weight Loss, Anti-aging, and Healing Your Own Body Fast for Beginners.* Thank you for taking the time to choose this book. This book is filled with all the subjects related to your water fasting needs. It will explain what water fasting is, and more importantly, how to do it. Each chapter will focus on an aspect specifically related to the outcomes of water fasting.

Chapter one is pretty much the main chapter of the book. It focuses on water fasting and will explain what it is and how it scientifically works. A brief history of both normal fasting and water fasting will be given to providing more insight into the process. Some basic health benefits and information will then be given as a way to tie in future chapters. The process of water fasting will then be explained in-depth. There will be specific directions on how to do it and what to expect.

Chapter two focuses specifically on autophagy. What

autophagy is and how it correlates with water fasting will be explained in this chapter. It will also explain the science behind autophagy and its health-related benefits. In addition, other ways to trigger the process will be listed that are not necessarily related to water fasting.

Chapter three is all about water fasting and weight loss. How weight loss and water fasting are related will be explained. It will also explain how water fasting ultimately helps the participant lose weight. A proof will be given for weight loss and how it works with water fasting.

Chapter four focuses on the anti-aging effects water fasting has on the inside and outside of the body. It relates to autophagy and explains how that causes anti-aging. The restorative properties will also be touched on and the real science behind these results.

Chapter five is all about the health benefits of water fasting. It will touch on both the mental and physical results that water fasting has on the body. All the restorative properties and diseases that fasting can treat will be listed and explained. The problems that can come from water fasting will also be listed.

There are plenty of books on this particular subject for sale both in stores and online. Thank you, once again, for choosing this specific book! Every effort was made to ensure the information in this book is as useful as possible. Hopefully, it is enjoyable and overall, very beneficial in whatever you hope to achieve through water fasting. So, please enjoy!

Water Fasting

FASTING IS a word which often brings many different thoughts to mind. Some might correlate the word with strict religious holidays while others may see it as a dietary fad. Fasting is defined as a process of not consuming food for long periods of time, even when the food is easily obtainable. It has a long and full history as it has been used for many different reasons throughout time. Most recently, water fasting has made its way into the spotlight of mainstream media because of its use in weight loss and numerous scientifically proven health benefits. Water fasting is a different take on a traditional fast as it only allows water to be regularly consumed. This being said, some regimens do allow certain types of coffees and teas to be consumed as well.

Recent studies that are focusing on fitness and weight have revealed the health benefits of water fasting. It has been revealed that this type of fast may assist in lowering certain types of chronic diseases. This means that a water fast can improve the chances of preventing heart disease and even cancer. Autophagy, the body's process of recycling old cells, can be triggered by doing water fasting. Autophagy has the ability to dispose of cells that may be cancerous and dangerous. This can be beneficial in renewing and healing the body's pre-existing healthy cells. At the end of the day, plenty of research has gone into the process of water fasting. This allows the participant to look into what medical experts are saying before even beginning the process. Research conducted on mice who participated in water fasting found positive results. The mice showed signs of improved blood pressure, a healthier body weight, and even the disappearing of rheumatoid arthritis symptoms. Science has shown that water fasting can be used for the benefit of the participant.

While water fasting may be most popular among the fitness and health community today, it also serves many other communities and purposes. Numerous religious organizations have a long and varied relationship with the process of water fasting. Some even use it today during special holidays and events like Ramadan, Lent, and Yom Kippur. Detoxing is also a popular dieting and health technique among those who do the water fasting diet. They use this process with the sole intent to flush their system and to clear their body of potentially harmful wastes. Sometimes, detoxing is used to clear the mind of stress and anxiety too. The process does not always have to be about the physical body and health.

Another portion of the community uses water fasting to improve their overall health and body. Some use this process for pre-existing conditions like chronic pain and even sudden and genetic conditions like heart disease. It has proven to be used successfully to treat and prevent potential illnesses and cancers. Even weight can be lost, thanks to water fasting. It can even assist in the surgical process of medical procedures. Water fasting is often recommended to people who will be undergoing surgical procedures in the near future. Doctors usually recommend 24-hour water fast to their patients before surgeries. This is to prevent the contents of the stomach from entering the airway which is a common effect of heavy amnesia. Water fasting has a variety of uses, all unique and beneficial for the health of the participating individual.

Despite these numerous reasons, most people in modern society choose to water fast for the health and weight loss benefits that come from the process. Several studies have proven that the beneficial process of water fasting can be used to lower the risk of cancers, heart diseases, and diabetes. That being said, water fasting also has a variety of health risks. It can be responsible for the worsening of gout, diabetes, chronic kidney disease, eating disorders, chronic migraines, and even heartburn.

Another type of diet called a 'Lemon Detox to cleanse,' was inspired by and based on water fasting. This is where the user only drinks a mixture of lemon juice, water, maple syrup, and cayenne pepper. The process lasts for several days and the concoction should be consumed several times a day. People often use this as an alternative for when they find water fasting boring or not effective enough. It is a beneficial and equally effective form of water fasting for those who want to try something new.

Those who choose to participate in the process of water fasting often do so for a variety of reasons. Whether it is used before a serious surgical operation or in the midst of a weight loss campaign, water fasting works. Those who want to improve their bodies and even their minds can find a solution in the water fasting process and its effects. It is an interesting process that boasts numerous health benefits and opportunities.

To understand the full impact and idealism of water fasting, one must first look at its historical origins. Traditional, non-water-based fasting has been present on this planet before humans even roamed it. In fact, even the earliest of the Earth's living creatures, including dinosaurs, would voluntarily fast during periods of stress or illness. Animals will still do this today in times of uneasiness or food shortages in their natural habitats. Fasting is a natural phenomenon shared by both humans and animals originally during times of tension and difficulty. It is even somewhat hard for historians to pinpoint when fasting first became popular among humans considering our long and varied history with the subject.

The earliest, primitive cultures and civilizations, like the

Mesopotamia, valued fasting for a variety of different reasons. Prior to a serious war or battle, these early people would fast as a way to prepare for the horrors of combat and warfare. They also used to fast as a coming of age ritual of sorts. This was when young participants would take part in a fast to prove their maturity and age. Early Native American tribes used to fast as a way to appease their angry polytheistic deities. They believed that this would help them prevent natural disasters and the threat of famine.

Fasting first became recognized as healthcare and therapy during the height of the Roman Empire. Numerous early great philosophers and healers, such as Plato, Socrates, and even Aristotle recommended fasting for its numerous healing properties and benefits. These early Greek philosophers and healers were among the first human beings to recognize that fasting was common amongst both humans and animals in states of distress or illness. They stated that it could be easily observed that when one is ill, they often don't wish to consume more food. It was viewed as a way for the body to naturally heal itself. For this reason, the early philosophers dubbed fasting, 'the physician within'. This means that fasting has always been a part of us and is as old as human nature itself.

This wasn't the only discovery the Greeks made when it came to fasting. In fact, they concluded that fasting is responsible for the improvement of cognitive abilities. They witnessed that after consuming overly large meals, their subjects were more likely to feel tired and irritable. It was proven that this is because blood is redirected to the stomach to aid in digestion, for that reason, making it more difficult to perform actions and sometimes even think logically.

These men were not alone in their discovery as fasting and its healing abilities spread to the western hemisphere. Philip Paracelsus, the founder of toxicology and one of the founding fathers of Western medicine, agreed with the statement that fasting is indeed 'the physician within'. Even the United States' own Founding Father, Ben Franklin, often recommended fasting and resting when it came to illnesses, disorders, and diseases. He made claims that it was indeed the absolute best way to heal.

Religion has always played a major role in the continuation and popularity of the practice of fasting. Jesus Christ, Buddha, and Muhammad were all rumored to be large supporters of fasting and its various effects. Religious organizations all around the world who were never even aware of each other's existence at the time adopted fasting. It was obviously well sought-after and thoroughly practiced. They used it not with the intent to harm or starve but to heal people's bodies, minds, and even their souls and spirits.

Buddhism supported the concept of fasting by encouraging followers to only consume food once every morning and to not eat again until the very next day. This religion was actually one of the first to adopt the concept of water fasting. Buddhist monks and followers would reportedly only drink water for days, sometimes even weeks on end without a single scrap of food. They credited their ability to do so to Buddha and his fundamental teachings.

Greek Orthodox Christians adopted a much more intense way to fast. Followers of this religious organization would often fast for upwards of 180 to 200 days a year. They would include forty days into their regimen for Lent, a holiday which honors Christ's forty days lost in the desert. The population of Greek Orthodox Christian in Crete was actually once considered the healthiest group of people in the Mediterranean by Dr. Ancel Keys.

Judaism valued fasting many times a year as a way to honor holy periods of time. Their most preferred and popular holiday for fasting is Yom Kippur, also known as the Day of Atonement. During this 25-hour period, participants would fast, pray intensively, and attend synagogue services.

Islam is the most associated religion with fasting because of the holy month of Ramadan which takes place in the ninth month of the Islamic calendar. Fasting was also encouraged to take place twice a week by the great prophet Muhammad. Ramadan differed from traditional methods of fasting as followers were not allowed to consume any liquids either. As they were only allowed to consume food while the sun was down, scientists noticed something interesting about their caloric intake: gorging on food after not eating all day actually showed signs of health benefits.

Despite the long history of fasting, a new and different type of fasting was introduced by Dr. Herbert Shelton in the 19th century. He claimed himself to be the first to discover the healing properties of water fasting. He wrote books over his achievement during the height of the Natural Hygiene Movement and even opened a school to teach the practice of water fasting. Dr. Shelton claimed he saved over 40,000 individual lives using the healing properties of water fasting. Unfortunately, he abused his power as a doctor which led to a negligent homicide charge. This occurred after one of his patients died due to starvation while following his fasting regimen. Despite this, he still practiced and promoted water fasting for the rest of his life.

It is clear that fasting has a varied and common history, and that it still plays a major role in health and religion today. It has shown to be a source of not only spiritual but also physical and mental healing all over the world. Water fasting has especially come quite a long way from the days of Buddha and Dr. Shelton. In the more modern era, the practice of water fasting is much more closely monitored and shows great health and healing benefits when done correctly.

The in-depth process of water fasting has become better researched and developed in the present years. It is now much easier to attempt and do so safely in the comfort of one's own home. The process of doing a water fast should be closely monitored for the best results.

Before one begins, they must evaluate the risks that come with water fasting. For example, exceeding the recommended limit of a three-day fasting period can come with health risks. Those who are too young or too old should not participate in water fasting either as this can pose serious health problems and risks. If you are under eighteen or an older adult, then you are highly discouraged from participating in the process of water fasting. Older adults who have fasted have shown signs of problems with their immune systems after finishing a fast. If you are under the weight limit for your age and sex, then you should definitely reconsider water fasting. Like all things, water fasting comes with risks and should be done in moderation. You should know your own body and its limits before taking part in the process of water fasting. It can be a beneficial process if done correctly. If not, then serious injury or even death may occur. It is highly suggested that you take the time to contact your doctor or healthcare professional before participating in water fast.

There are several types of people who should not participate in fasting for the good of their own health. This includes the aforementioned minors, elders, and those who are underweight. Those who have an eating disorder like bulimia, anorexia, or a binge-eating disorder should not participate in any type of fast, including water-based. Mothers who are breastfeeding or pregnant are highly discouraged from participation in this process. Anyone with a severe heart problem or Type one diabetes should refrain from attempting a water fast. Those who are susceptible to severe and chronic migraines should not participate as it has the potential to only worsen the effects. Anyone planning on donating blood or receiving a blood transfusion should postpone water fast until a healthcare professional or a doctor recommends that it is safe for them to begin. If the potential participant is taking any type of prescribed medication, they should speak to their doctor or a medical professional before beginning a fast. As always, a doctor should be consulted before making any large dietary changes, such as water fasting, to ensure positive and desired results.

If you have never experienced a fast of any type, you should not just jump right in. Instead, you should try a one-day water fast to test the effects the process may have on your body. If any problems arise or the participant feels uncomfortable with the fast, then they can stop at any time and not continue with the process of water fasting. If the water fast goes well then, intermittent water fast should be the next goal. This is when a fast goes on and off for a few days at a time. Both of these processes will prepare the body for a longer more intense water fast. It is best to choose which one you think will work best for you and your body's health.

To begin, it is wise for you to plan ahead your potential fasting experience. As the participant, you should choose a time during which you are mostly inactive to participate in water fasting. It would not be a good idea to attend work or school or do exercise while fasting due to vitiligo (light-headedness). You would not want to risk the possibility of passing out due to these activities. Choose a week during which you have time off as you will need time to prepare before, and time to recover after. Taking this into consideration, a participant should feel safe and relaxed while fasting.

The length of time you should take to water fast is not set in stone. This does not mean it can just last for weeks, though. In fact, most licensed medical and healthcare professionals recommend that water fasts should only last between 24-hours and three days. A medical professional or licensed doctor should be contacted before taking on a three day or a longer fast to prevent medical complications. Three days should also be the limit on participation at any time over can cause serious and even severe medical problems to occur.

It is also often recommended that water fasting is to be done in the company of others who can properly supervise you and your health. Those who are planning on participating in a water fast to alleviate, or even attempt to cure a medical condition, should have a supervisor. Water fasting can be dangerous to some, even those who believe that they are perfectly healthy and can do a water fast with no problems have experienced injuries. Albeit, the danger usually comes from fainting due to standing up too fast, but it is still a potential health threat. Those who are considered seriously overweight or underweight should only participate in a water fast with a supervisor. If you have struggled with controlling your calorie intake and overall weight, then some challenges may need to be overcome with the help of a supervisor. Some can get emotional with the concept of food and eating. If you are worried about your state of mental health while fasting, then a supervisor is highly recommended. Eating disorders can arise from participating in the water fast while overweight.

Some might be wondering about the best way to find a supervisor and who the supervisor should be. It is always a good idea to experience a water fast with the help of a supervisor, especially if it's your first. It is wise to have someone who is an expert or has prior experience as they can walk you through the process and alleviate potential concerns and anxieties. Professionals who are involved in the world of dieting and fasting are familiar with health issues that may arise and often know the proper way to treat them. They can also tailor the experience especially to you and your body based on your health history and future concerns. They may even advise that water fast would not be wise for you to participate in at all. Most practitioners experienced with water fasting may recommend that you visit them at their office or clinic. However, a select few can call or video chat with you from the comfort of your own home while in the middle of water fast. Some may also recommend that based on your prior medical history or current condition that you instead visit a doctor while water fasting. A doctor can also be a type of supervisor while partaking in a water fast. Despite this, they may not be thoroughly experienced with the process of water fasting as well as the emotional influence behind it. It is pretty much up to you to decide what will be the best for your personal health and well-being.

If you instead choose to participate in the water fast without supervision, then it is wise to know your own body and to prepare ahead of time. This isn't too difficult as most participants choose to water fast on their own and do so successfully. It is only recommended that you are supervised by a fasting professional. In the few weeks before beginning a water fast, the participant should mentally and physically prepare. These periods can be tiring and draining both the mind and body. It is not wise to just begin week-long water fast tomorrow or even the day after. Instead, try going one day with only small amounts of food like rice or fruit first. Intermittent fasting is also a popular way to begin. An example of this would be water fasting one day a week every week leading up to the main fast. This can help you better understand your body's relationship with hunger and food. If you have a habit of consuming unhealthy fast food and junk food quite often it will be more difficult to begin water fast. You may want to attempt a cleansing detox a month beforehand to flush your system of all that toxic food.

In the few days leading up to a water fast, it is best to prepare. This can be done by eating proportional amounts of food beforehand. It should not deviate from the participant's normal amount of food intake. Instead, try foods that can provide high energy and that are relatively healthy. It is not wise to do water fasting when you're ill, so if a cold arises a fast can always be rescheduled. It is also encouraged to reschedule a water fast when the participant feels just tired or not up to it. Finally, consider beginning a fast slowly. One can do this by slowly cutting or reducing daily meals and snacks. This makes it easier on the body to adapt.

When the participant finally has everything ready and feels confident, then it should be time to begin. First off, one may use large amounts of water to try and compensate for the hunger they are feeling. They should instead take in the normal amount of water they usually would and try not to overdrink. The usual doctor recommended amount is a healthy two to three liters or quarts of water a day. It's about the same amount, just different units of measurement. It is wise to only drink when thirsty as to not overdrink. Over-drinking can make one sick and should be avoided at all costs.

The type of water you choose for a water fast plays an important role in the process. Distilled water is often the most recommended drink for water fasters. Despite its healing properties and benefits, this specific type of water is not recommended for everyday non-fasting consumption. It is only recommended for its noticeably increased ability to bind to and prevent toxins. All in all, it is wise to only drink distilled water over the period of a water fast.

When a water fast is first begun, it can be an incredibly difficult and even painful process. After all, the first few days after a water fast begins are often credited by participants as the most intense. Going without food can have a difficult emotional toll on the mind. The detoxification process of water fasting can also be somewhat uncomfortable and even painful. It is normal to feel irritable, fatigued, and sickly throughout, and even after a water fast. If you do feel dizzy, weak, or nauseous at any time throughout the fast then just know that that is also quite normal. However, if these symptoms become too intense, it is important to eat. If you also begin to feel disoriented or confused, this is not normal. It is important to stop and contact a doctor or medical professional, but do keep in mind that a few days after a water fast has begun it becomes much easier to handle. Discomfort often disappears almost completely, and the gnawing sensation of hunger disappears, as well. This is because of a natural process which is commonly known as ketosis. Ketosis is when the body begins to replace the nourishment, which was once caused by food, with the internal burning of the body's fat cells. Doctor Joel Fuhrman has recorded that this process kicks in at about 48 hours for women and 72 hours for men. However, the time period during which the body is under the state of ketosis varies from person to person, so it is always wise to converse with your doctor or healthcare professional before beginning. When the feeling of hunger returns, then it is recommended that the water fast has ended as this is when the body gets truly desperate for nourishment.

Whether you choose to participate in a water fast for religion or health, it should be a time of rejuvenation and relaxation. Remember to spend most of the time sitting and to not participate in any vigorous exercise during a water fast. This will help conserve energy. All in all, water fasting is a process which requires personal attention and self-love. You must honor the process, the rest, and the bodily awareness that goes into water fasting. It is best to listen to your body and honor what it needs and says. The final goal should be one of healing and positive change. It is also necessary to know when to stop. If you feel as though you cannot take it anymore, it is okay to quit. There is no shame in interpreting your body's signals and needs for the better. All in all, it is a bonding process between you and your own body and should be treated as such.

When it is time for the water fast to reach an end, don't immediately begin eating or eat too much. Instead, gradually build up meals or try smoothies so the body can adapt. Attempting to begin eating too much immediately after a fast can result in death. This is due to something called Refeeding syndrome. It's when the body undergoes potentially fatal changes in fluid and electrolytes too rapidly. Just make sure you take your time, and in return, your stomach will thank you. Expect to feel tired and fatigued a few days after ending the water fast. The body needs time to bounce back from the lack of incoming nutrients. It will usually take the same amount of days as the fast lasts to fully recover. Remember to not immediately start eating afterward, especially if the food of choice is unhealthy. You may regain all the weight you lost. After you've finished, rejoice and appreciate a healthier you! Even if it was only for a day, a water fast can be difficult to do and is something to be celebrated.

You now know how to do a water fast and what it can entail

for your health, but you do not yet know the specifics of the way it works on the body. For those who have specific medical conditions, it's important to understand what fasting does to your body. And those who are purely curious or nervous deserve to know too. The effects of water fasting are important to know for those who are committed to it.

Water fasting can help with both life-threatening and cosmetic ailments and illnesses. Those who have participated in water fasts have reported little, but still amazing effects that are just results of the process. Water fast can be reportedly used to clear the appearance of something small, like moles. Achy muscles and bones which have been present for years are said to be miraculously healed with a couple days of water fasting. Even weird blotches of skin are gone practically overnight thanks to the miracle that is water fasting. These are only the small effects that come from water fasting. It has a variety of much larger healing and prevention benefits.

Those with high blood pressure would find the effects of water fasting extremely beneficial. Extensive research has proven that supervised water fasts can greatly lower the blood pressure of those with naturally high blood pressure. In 2002, a study was conducted to determine whether or not patients with borderline high blood pressure could be treated with water fasting. A total of 68 subjects were selected for testing. For nearly fourteen straight days they participated in a water fast under strict medical supervision. They were tested at the end of the trial and all their blood pressure results showed major improvements. By the end of the 14-day water fast, 82 percent of the test subjects reported their blood pressure levels returning to a normal amount. A year later, a different experiment with a similar hypothesis published their findings. This time it was an amount of 174 total test subjects. This group of individuals did a water fast for 10 to 11 total days. When the water fast ended, 90 percent of the participants were surprised to find that their blood pressure dropped to the limited amount used to diagnose blood pressure. Unfortunately, scientists don't know yet if a 24-hour to three days water fast would have the same effects. This means that this type of extended water fast can only be possible in a controlled environment.

Water fasting can also improve the symptoms in those who possess insulin and leptin sensitivity. Both insulin and leptin are crucial hormones which affect the body's metabolism. Insulin's main job in the body is to assist in the storage of nutrients that have migrated in from the bloodstream. Leptin plays a different, yet similar in the body's digestive system. Its primary function is to make you feel full and to prevent overeating. Several different researchers have ulti-mately concluded that participating in a water fast could help your body by making it more sensitive to both insulin and leptin. This great increase in sensitivity makes these hormones in your body even more effective. By developing a high sensitivity to insulin and its effects, your body becomes more efficient at reducing high blood sugar. Being more sensitive to the leptin hormone means different health results. This can help your body process hunger signals much more effectively. In turn, this process can help lower the chance of obesity.

There are several chronic diseases which can be prevented by the process of water fasting. Several scientific studies and research have pointed to the fact that water fasting can help improve in lowering the risk of several chronic diseases. Some of these diseases are diabetes, cancer, and heart disease. Animal studies have revealed similar impressive and miraculous results. These studies revealed the animal's heart to be protected from radicals after water fasting. Radicals that are free within the body are unstable and unpredictable molecules that can cause harm and damage to otherwise healthy cells. Radicals are listed as one of the main causes as chronic diseases. Similar studies done on animals involving water fasting have revealed similar healthy results. These studies showed that water fasting can help in the suppression of genes which have been known to cause the growth of cancer cells. In those who already have cancer, water fasting can help improve several side effects listed that come with chemotherapy. A study held in 2013 focused on 30 healthy adults. They were told to do water fasting for 24 total hours with somewhat interesting results. When their water fasting ended, their blood showed significantly lower levels of cholesterol and triglycerides. This effectively means that their risk of heart disease lowered. Overall, water fasting can be used to treat and prevent life-threatening chronic diseases.

While there are many health benefits that come with water fasting and its processes, not all effects are physical. Most who participate in water fasting report an overall improved mental health by the end of the fast. Science has backed this up too, often crediting autophagy to the distressing process which comes from water fasting. Those who participate in these types of fasts often report feeling a lot better during and after the fast. They claim that it helps manage anxiety, depression, and stress in a healthier way. The thought of them "doing something healthy" reportedly helps during this emotionally fulfilling process. There is often an emotional and physical high reported with water fasting by its participants. Some even claim that it overweighs the gnawing hunger that usually comes with the strenuous process. It helps both the body and mind feel not only better, but healthier as well.

All in all, water fasting is a marvelous process with a host of benefits. This type of fasting has a varied history that began with Buddha's teachings. It played a large role in the Natural Hygiene Movement and was a health favorite of Dr. Herbert Shelton. It has greatly improved in recent years with new research happening all the time. Water fasting has a strict process which must be closely followed for the best health results. If done so, it can prevent heart disease and cancer. It aids in numerous healing processes, like autophagy. It is a health craze that is sure to stick around.

Autophagy

AUTOPHAGY IS A BODILY process which is often correlated with water fasting. It is a process which has much better weight loss results compared to that of juice cleanses and detox diets. Autophagy is a natural process during which the body cleanses itself. It's when the old cells throughout your body are broken down and then recycled. To specify, the process is largely responsible for the removal of old cell membranes, organelles, and miscellaneous types of cell-based debris. The waste is then sent via the autophagosomes to specific organelles within the body to break them down. For example, some are sent to lysosomes because they contain a digestive enzyme which can completely destroy the old cells. Some compare it to the body eating itself, too. This process is something you can actually train yourself to do using multiple techniques including water fasting.

This unique type of cell was first discovered by a Belgian

scientist in 1963. His name was Christian de Duve, and he was a biochemist from Belgium. This man was actually responsible for naming the cell, autophagy. However, its real importance and actual purpose went unknown for about 30 years. In the 1990s, Japanese researchers finally found out what autophagy did within the body. This was discovered after observing the cell function in yeast. It was at this time one Japanese researcher unlocked the true potential of autophagy. Yoshinori Ohsumi was praised highly for his discovery. In 2016, he was awarded a Nobel Prize in Physiology or Medicine. It is because of this reason that many people trust autophagy and what it can do within the body. Thanks to his research, a whole new way of healthy living has been opened up for those who like to do water fasting.

Autophagy literally translates to "self-eating". It actually works in a very similar way to the process of cleaning out your house. Your cells begin autophagy by creating a special type of membrane whose sole purpose is to hunt down cells. It often targets specific cells within the body that are dead, diseased, malfunctioning, or worn out. It then consumes these rotting cells all the while stripping them for sections within the cell that still may hold value and use.

Finally, the resulting molecules are used to provide energy to the body or transform into a completely new part. An example of this would be amino acids which came from an old, worn cell. These amino acids could be transferred to the liver where it will be used in the creation of glucose. It can also just be added as extra support to healthy proteins throughout the body. Autophagy is practically a way of making the body act like a well-oiled machine that disposes of faulty and dangerous cells. It is credited for reducing the chances of tumors and other cancerous growths and preventing metabolic dysfunctions.

One of the main reasons autophagy happens is because cells need to be relieved of stressful conditions. This process is also responsible for a large part of cellular development and differentiation. Autophagy has also been proven to help in basic immunity and prevent numerous diseases. It does this by assisting in blocking invading pathogens. Overall, these benefits improve not only the cell's system but also the bodies. However, too much autophagy can also be bad and can cause stress on the body. There is a balance to autophagy production within the body. Doctors and other healthcare professionals recommend a balanced amount of eating and fasting instead of just dieting. As always, everything in moderation.

Autophagy is sometimes confused for a process called apoptosis. This is a process during which an entire cell is destroyed, instead of recycled. These cells' main job is to completely dispose of problematic cells. However, this doesn't always work to the body's benefits. This is because apoptosis has a history of accidentally contributing to diseases like cancer and neurodegeneration. Cancer is when cells multiply out of control and neurodegeneration is the exact opposite. It is when cells begin to die off too quickly.

Autophagy does something like this, but not as intense. It only destroys cells to recycle them and to make cell parts.

The reason why autophagy is not always active is that of eating. When we eat, autophagy comes to a pause within our bodies which is why we usually don't notice it working. This is why water fast is a great way to encourage the process of autophagy. Water fasting provides caloric restrictions as well as other perks that trigger autophagy to work. If you were to only consume a fatty diet, then autophagy would happen all the time. It doesn't take that much food to stop autophagy either which is why water fasting is an ideal way to promote it.

A crucial key regulator with autophagy is mTOR. This is a specific type of energy-based enzyme that is responsible for the transfer of specific phosphate groups. This is better known as the process which changes the ATP (adenosine triphosphate) into ADP (adenosine diphosphate). ATP is responsible for energy within the body, and it also keeps you on your feet and feeling energized. MTOR's main job is the management of energy within the body. This would include process like cell growth, protein synthesis, and of course, autophagy. To summarize, mTOR disrupts the process of autophagy during activation. Autophagy increases incredibly when mTOR isn't active. The only way to prevent its activation is to perform a water fast. However, when you do eat, mTOR is active and so, amino acid and insulin levels increase tremendously. Scientific research has proved these claims too.

A recent study found that eight healthy men who completed a 72 hour fast had lower levels of mTOR activation. This makes sense evolutionarily speaking. When food is common and there is no possibility of starving, the body understands this and adapts to these terms. However, just like autophagy, too much mTOR can have dangerous and damaging results on the body. Increasing your body's amount of mTOR is great for aspects pertaining to muscle gain and cognitive power. Decreasing it has different results like decreasing the risk of cancer and inflammation both in the body and on the surface of the skin. This also increases your overall lifespan. While normal amounts of mTOR are all well and good, too much can be severe. An unusually high amount of mTOR can lead to obesity, type 2 diabetes, cancer, depression, and sometimes even acne.

The way to activate mTOR is through the opposite of water fasting. A successful activation can be achieved by simply eating normal amounts. Eating is not the only activator though. Exercise plays a big part in mTOR activation and so does hormones like testosterone and even insulin. If you wish to deactivate mTOR then a water fast or even consuming protein is highly recommended by doctors and healthcare professionals. There are other ways to decrease mTOR supply as well. These are things like aspirin, alcohol, and ketogenic diets. Different types of nutrients like Epigallocatechin gallate (which can be found in green tea), caffeine, Curcumin, and Resveratrol. Certain types of drugs are also responsible for inhibiting mTOR activation like

Metformin. There are many different ways to activate and inhibit mTOR. What's best to take away from this is that this kind of process must be attempted in moderation. Water fasting is recommended as the best way to achieve this perfect harmony.

Studies have also shown that the process also heals and improves inflammation within the body and immunity to disease. In 2012, a group of scientists engineered a few selected rats in a specific way. These rats were incapable of experiencing autophagy and therefore didn't have access to the effects it usually has on the body. This caused them to develop a heavier weight and a more fatigued demeanor. They also showed signs of a higher cholesterol count and impaired brain function. To sum it up, autophagy is extremely important to our health.

This process has many health benefits. In fact, autophagy can assist in the quick repair of injuries, whether that is a broken bone or a paper cut. It also assists your brain with improving cognitive thinking and function. This means that it helps you focus on and understand more complicated subjects. Those who enjoy fitness most likely already know of autophagy and its benefits. It assists in the process of gaining muscle mass as well as shedding a few pounds. Autophagy can even be credited to helping with everyday tasks like movement and respiration. Sometimes, these activities can cause damage to the body even if it's minor. Autophagy is the process meant to repair your body and keep it in working order.

Autophagy has often been called the fountain of youth by health gurus and licensed experts alike. Many have credited this as the reason they look so young for their age. This is because it possesses the ability to slow the aging process. In fact, the founder of autophagy, Nobel Prize winner Yoshinori Ohsumi, was the one who discovered autophagy's ability to turn back the clock on age. After all, aging is just the result of accumulating dysfunctional proteins and organelles within our once healthy cells. Cells can be kept healthier longer, thanks to autophagy and its ability to clean the house and dispose of unwanted cells. Anti-aging is not the only benefit of autophagy which can be triggered by water fasting.

The process of water fasting can also encourage autophagy to help with improving the brain's health and cognitive ability. Autophagy can help the metabolic process in supporting the brain's ability to stay healthy and high-performing. Through autophagy, many processes can be improved within the body. One of these are the numerous circulating levels of many neurotrophic factors which autophagy increases. These factors are biomolecules that support neuron health as well as their overall survival and growth. This process comes with many beneficial results. One of these benefits is the increased openness for learning and concentration. Another is an overall decrease in stress and anxiety. This process also supports an increased amount of cognitive energy.

Autophagy can also help with a decrease of inflammation

and oxidative stress. This occurs when damaged and old cells are removed through the process of autophagy. It can also help with the process of stimulating endogenous antioxidants. Basically, both of these different functions help with the improvement of the brain's ability and function. Not only does autophagy assists now, but it also has effects which are more present in the future. Water fasting and autophagy have been proven to reduce the long-term effects of neuronal dysfunctions that come from diseases like Alzheimer's and Parkinson's.

The body's composition can also be healed via the effects of autophagy from water fasting. Most people often blame weight on calorie intake by the individual. Even nutritionists and dietitians get confused by this myth. However, recent scientific studies have shown that this belief is not completely true. The body's weight is actually based on the hormonal state of the individual. Autophagy is responsible for increasing insulin sensitivity and adiponectin levels during a water fast.

These two key hormones have quite a lot to do with weight gain and loss. They determine if fat gets used for energy instead of just sitting. They also decide whether or not incoming calories are to be fat or if they are to be immediately implemented somewhere within the body. Even after a water fast is completed, the effects of autophagy continue, meaning this process can go on for quite some time. Yes, calories will decrease during a water fast, but it is only when the fast is happening. The hormonal changes will instead stay active within the body for weeks, sometimes even months.

Autophagy can improve your digestive system and its assist with the natural process. Water fasting allows the digestive system to go into a sort of natural reset mode. During this process, the gastrointestinal tract gets a chance to relax for a bit. This means that intestinal inflammation is reduced which is beneficial for your digestive system. Another process this encourages is improved motility which is when the gastrointestinal muscles are contracted to aid in the digestion process. Both assist in the process of nutrient absorption and a better quality of waste.

Besides water fasting, there are numerous ways to encourage autophagy within your body. However, it is the most successful and reliable way to trigger autophagy. Despite this, autophagy can be found anywhere within the body and works with a variety of systems. A few recent scientific studies have found evidence to support autophagy working within the liver and brain. Data can be found connecting these cases and proving their success. First, the level of the activity within the autophagy process can be measured by counting the interior cellular organelles. These organelles are called autophagosomes and their job is the handling of dysfunctional protein degradation. These will increase in amount when autophagy is triggered by the act of a water fast. A study that examined liver cells discovered that the total amount of autophagosomes increased when the participant was doing a water fast. The amount originally increased 300 percent after a 24-hour water fast. After 48 total hours of fasting, that amount increased by another 30 percent.

Some studies focusing on brain cells found similar interesting results. These studies also focused on autophagosomes located within brain cells and found metabolic markers which proved that autophagy was, in fact, being stimulated in the brain. This increase in active autophagy showed a peak in metabolic markers between 24 and 36 hours. This means that fasting for longer periods of time can prove amazing health results and benefits. However, studies have found that after 36 total hours of water fasting, the amount of changes seems to even out instead of constantly increasing.

The entire process of autophagy and the benefits that come with it may sound quite enticing. Unfortunately, some may not be able to participate in a water fast due to various reasons like health, weight, and many more. Instead, there are other ways to trigger autophagy that don't include fasting.

One way to promote autophagy is exercise. Some can find exercise an incredibly daunting task, especially doing it often enough to promote autophagy. This is for a reason, of course, as exercise is supposed to put stress on the body. Working out can actually damage muscles (Don't worry, it's normal.) by causing microscopic tears in the muscle lining.

This is why you're so sore and physically weak after a tedious work out session.

The tears in the muscles are then quickly healed by the body which in turn makes them stronger and more resistant to tearing and damage. Exercise is actually a way of helping the body cleanse. A study held in 2012 actually helped with connecting autophagy to exercise. They were bred to have glowing green autophagosomes which would be monitored when the mice participated in the exercise. After running on a treadmill for a total of 30 minutes, the mice's cells were recycling themselves at a much faster rate. The rate continued at a steady pace for the total of 80 minutes that they ran. It is recommended that for the best results, intense exercise sessions should be attempted.

A different way to promote autophagy besides the traditional water fast would be lowering your general carb intake. This process can be done by practically anyone as it's pretty much a type of diet. Ketosis is a new type of diet that holds a place among bodybuilders and those who want to prevent aging and its effects. This method supports taking in as little carbohydrates as possible. Therefore the body has no use but to use fat as fuel instead. This diet is not like other diets as you don't have to deviate much from your meal plan. Although, sugar is definitely not encouraged with this diet. This process is praised for its ability to assist in weight loss while still leaving valuable muscle mass intact. It can also help the body in similar health-related ways to water fasting. There is scientific evidence supporting that lowering carb intake can prevent cancer and tumors, lower diabetes risk, and protect the brain against epilepsy and other related brain disorders. In fact, a recent scientific study showed that children who do the ketosis diet have a 50 percent overall reduction in seizures.

Understanding the benefits of autophagy

The benefits of autophagy are truly remarkable. Many of the healing benefits that you can get with a water fast come because you start the process of autophagy throughout your body. There are actually a lot of benefits that can come with autophagy and research suggests that some of the most important benefits of this process include:

1. Provides your cells with the molecular building blocks and energy they need
2. Recycles the damaged aggregates, organelles, and proteins that build up in the body
3. Regulates the functions of the mitochondria in the cells, which can produce a ton of energy but can be damaged when oxidative stress occurs in the body
4. Clears out the damaged endoplasmic reticulum and peroxisomes
5. Protects the nervous system and can encourage the growth of brain and nerve cells - Autophagy is able to help improve the neuroplasticity, brain structure, and cognitive function in individuals who give it time to occur.

6. Supports the growth of heart cells and is a great way to protect yourself against heart disease
7. Can enhance the immune system because it is able to eliminate intracellular pathogens
8. Defends against toxic proteins that are going to be the root cause of many diseases in the body
9. Can protect how stable DNA is
10. Prevents against any damage to healthy organs and tissues in a process that is known as necrosis
11. Can potentially help an individual fight off a bunch of different illnesses, neurodegenerative diseases, and fights cancer

Now, you will find that there are different kinds of autophagy. This can include chaperone-mediated autophagy, microautophagy, and macroautophagy. The macroautophagy is the one that we are going to hear about the most and is usually the one that people will talk about when they bring up autophagy.

Humans are not the only ones who are going to benefit from this process. In fact, autophagy is something that has been observed in many different species including mammals, flies, worms, plants, mold, and yeast. Most of the research that has been done concerning autophagy will involve yeast and rats. And a minimum of 32 autophagy-related genes were identified by genetic screening studies. Research continues to show that these processes are important responses in the body through many species for stress and starvation.

How to induce autophagy

If you want to get all of the benefits that come with autophagy and you want to be able to get the dead and damaged cells replaced in your body, so you feel better than ever before, then it is important to know how to induce autophagy. When does this autophagy occur? This is a process that is going to be active in all cells, but it will increase by quite a bit in response to stress or nutrient deprivation, which can be either starvation or fasting.

What this means is that you can use some good stressors like fasting or exercise to boost the autophagic processes. Both of these are going to be linked with a lot of benefits including weight control, longevity, and the prevention of many diseases that are associated with age.

The main way that you can induce autophagy in the body is through fasting. This includes intermittent fasting and water fasting. Fasting is a simple concept for you to work with. You simply need to abstain from eating for a certain amount of time, usually between one to ten days depending on what your goals are and your overall health when you get started. Some types of fasts allow you to have tea or coffee, but for a water fast, make sure that you don't add these in.

The next question here is how long you need to be on a fast in order to reach autophagy. Studies show that a fast that goes between 24 to 48 hours is going to give you the strongest effects. If you want to go on a water fast each week or on a more regular basis, then this length of time is probably the best to choose. As a beginner, you may want to start out with lower time limits, so going between 12 to 36 hours at a time can be a good way to get started.

While you are on the water fast, you will give the body a break from all the unhealthy foods, stresses, and other toxins that you are bringing into your life. Even a few days can make a big difference in when autophagy can occur, and how many benefits that you can get from it. You will quickly find that going through a fast, one that is a few days long at least can be one of the fastest ways to enter into this process.

In addition to going on a fast, exercise can help you to induce autophagy. Remember that you shouldn't do the exercise when you are on a fast, but if you want some help keeping the process of autophagy going even after the fast is done, then going on an exercise routine can provide you with the benefits that you are looking for. Research has been able to show recently that exercise will induce autophagy in many of the organs that are involved in metabolic regulation, such as the adipose tissue, pancreas, liver, and muscles.

While exercise is considered a very important thing to do to improve your health, it is considered a form of stress because it goes through and breaks down the tissues in your body, causing them to be repaired and then grow back stronger than ever before. It's not entirely sure how much exercise you need to go through in order to boost the autophagic process, but research does seem to suggest that doing a more intense form of exercise can be the most beneficial for seeing these results.

When it comes to the cardiac and skeletal muscle tissues, doing just 30 minutes of exercise can be enough to induce this process. If you go through just a small fast of a day, you may be able to do some exercise while fasting, but remember that for the longer fasts, you should be careful and not overdo it with the exercise, even considering just sitting back and not doing any exercise until the fast is all done.

Weight Loss

IT IS VERY MUCH possible to go through and use the water fast while also losing weight at the same time. Many people decide to go on a water fast that lasts up to seven days in order to help them lose weight quickly and even to prepare them for a diet plan that will start after they are done. There are a lot of ways that you are going to see weight loss when you go on a water fast, and you will actually be amazed at the results that you see.

The good news about water fasting is you will actually be able to lose weight in the process. There is a lot of talk out there about starvation mode and how it can mess with your metabolism, but if you make sure that you do the fast in the proper manner, and you don't go on the fast too long, you will be able to see some amazing results.

When you are practicing a water fast, there are going to be four main benefits that come from doing this process. These four benefits include diet program, therapy, detox, and metabolism booster. All of these can help you to lose weight faster and more efficiently than you can with any of the other methods for dieting and weight loss that you will see. Let's take a look at these four main benefits and how they will affect the results that you get.

Diet program

There are a lot of different diet plans that you are going to see on the market. Most of these programs are going to spend their time bombarding you with lots of myths and facts in the hopes of being able to get you to purchase their program rather than another one. However, one of the most effective diet programs out there that you can use is an occasional fast. There are numerous health benefits, and these alone can put a lot of other diet programs to shame. And since you don't have to spend any money, or make a lot of life adjustments, in order to get this started, when you start with the weight loss diet program of fasting, you will also be able to lose a ton of weight. The first reason for this is that this kind of fast forces the body to stop relying on the steady source of carbs it usually does for energy for a short amount of time while you are fasting. Instead, the body will rely on fat to keep you going. Through this process, you will be able to lose weight because you are getting rid of a lot of the extra fat that is accumulating in your body.

Since you are spending your time drinking just pure water, which doesn't have any calories in it, this means that for the length of your fast, you are going to go without any calories. That alone means that you aren't going to gain weight because more calories are being burned than you are taking in. This process is also going to trigger the tapping of adipose tissue for energy, which results in you shedding off fat and excess weight.

The second reason that you could lose weight is sometimes more complicated to understand. Water fasting is able to trigger the removal of body wastes, including salt. As these wastes are naturally flushed out of the body, the extra water that has been trapped in the body will go out as well. This flushing out of extra water weight can help you to see more weight loss than ever before.

Therapy

Throughout history, the process of fasting has been something that was used as a therapeutic practice. People who regularly went and practiced this believe that fasting is able to strengthen the body, the mind, and the soul. Since this is the case, it means that going on a water fast could, in turn, become a holistic form of therapy for the body to enjoy.

Not only is this practice therapeutic when it comes to the benefits that it provides to the body, but it also has the ability to change the way that you start to look at yourself. Fasting has been a life-changing process for many people. You may feel healthier and happier, you may start to appreciate all of the great things that your body is able to do, and you will really enjoy some of the changes that occur in all forms within the body during a water fast.

In addition, water fasting can be very therapeutic for the body because it is going to clean you from the inside out. This will be talked about a bit more in the following section about detoxification, but this detox is going to do a lot of wonders for the body. Even just a few days on this can really clean out the body and make you feel lighter and happier as a whole.

Water fasting can also provide some therapy for the mind. This is because it takes some effort and a higher state of mind in order to accomplish this kind of fast, especially if you go on one for a longer period of time. Fasting means that you would need to take better control over some of the external factors in your life, such as your hunger, in order to see the results that you are looking for.

And finally, water fasting can be therapeutic for the soul. This is important because it can help you to bring in a posi-tive aura and get rid of the negative aura around you. This is going to hold onto the answer of why people throughout history fast for a variety of religious reasons.

When you add in all of this therapy to your life, you are naturally going to feel better than ever before. And all of this can lead to making you lose weight easier than ever before.

Detox

If you have spent any time looking at the latest trends and

fads with weight loss, you have heard about the process of detoxification. While the market has a lot of different options that were created in order to help your body get rid of all the bad stuff, you will find that fasting is still considered the best and more effective detoxifier.

While the other ways of fasting can be effective on occasion, water fasting is going to be a natural and effective way to detoxify the whole body, and the results can be seen in just a few days. In addition, it is free to get started. As long as you have some water around you, you are going to see the results without a lot of expensive gadgets and tools to make it happen.

The cool thing about water is that it is the most powerful detoxifier in the world. It is able to clear out every toxin that is able to get into the body, and then it will flush them out as urine and stool. And then, because you are in a state of fasting, you will be able to trigger the body to start healing.

The energy that you would, otherwise, devote over to your gastrointestinal tract to heal you and deal with the foods that you commonly eat, can now be moved over to your immune system while you are on the fast. This helps you to not only clear things out but can give the immune system a little break and an added boost to keep you healthy. And then the physiologic functions for excreting wastes, that are done by the colon, lymphatics, kidney, and liver will be restored with the help of water.

A metabolism booster

It is believed and hypothesized by many medical experts that the way we eat is going to have a big effect on the way that our metabolism is able to work. This can go either way. If we eat healthy foods with lots of nutrients and eat the right amounts, then it is going to have a positive effect on your metabolism. However, if you have a poor diet and don't fill your body with the foods that it needs, it could lead to a lot of metabolic problems, including diabetes and other digestive issues.

Fasting is a good way to get your metabolism back on track. It will help to get that metabolism back to its optimal performance. It can also help to trigger some of the fat burning mechanisms that are inside the body. In normal eating, you would rely on carbs and sugars to provide you with the nutrients that you need because these are common in the foods that you eat, and they are often in ready supply. However, during a fast or another prolonged absence of food, the body naturally starts to turn towards the stored fat in the body to make up the energy that you need to survive.

Once you have been able to turn on the fat metabolism, putting on weight can become more and more difficult. At the same time, fasting would be able to correct a lot of the statistics of your metabolism. Pathologic metabolic factors, such as excessive cravings and insulin resistance would be regulated with the help of a fast. And finally, the speed and the health of your metabolism is going to be increased just by the fact that your digestive organs start to run clean and healthy.

All of this can work to help you lose weight. First, you're going to lose weight because the body starts to rely more on burning through the fat, rather than carbs when you are on the fast. In addition to this, your organs are now cleaning themselves out and working more efficiently, and it makes sense that you will be able to lose a lot of weight in the process. And when the metabolism works better and can speed up, the weight is going to feel like it is just melting off.

The types of weight loss while on a water fast

When it comes to losing weight on your water fast, there are actually a few things that are going on. We will talk about the five main causes of weight loss, which may help to explain why you are able to see results so quickly when you go on this kind of fast. Some of the most common reasons that you may see a lot of weight loss with a good water fast includes:

Water weight

Even though this kind of fast is all about drinking a ton of water, this can actually do some wonders when it comes to helping you get rid of the extra water weight that sticks around your body. No matter what fears you have about water fasting, you should never be afraid to drink lots of water throughout the fast. In fact, drinking as much water as you can during this process can help you to stay hydrated and can keep your metabolism working properly.

Many times, the weight that you lose during those first few

days will come because of the water that is sticking around the body. Being able to release this can help you to lose weight in no time at all. Often, the body holds onto water because of a variety of reasons (and some of those will be discussed as we keep going through this chapter). Once you fill up and make sure that you get plenty of water, the body will be more likely to drop the water weight, and you will see a lot of weight drop off in no time.

Fat weight loss

Even if you go on a fast that is just a day or two long, you will be able to lose some weight, thanks to the fat that is burned during that time. Traditionally, the body is going to rely on sugars like glucose to provide it with energy. Glucose is an easy form of energy and most of the American diet is full of it, but glucose is not very efficient as a form of fuel. What this means is that often we don't burn all of the glucose that we consume, even if we feel hungry for more, and this extra gets stored as body fat and extra weight.

When you go on a fast, especially one that is longer than a day or two, you take away that easy source of glucose. The body has to search around for some other fuel source to keep it going. During the first few days, you may feel tired and worn out because of this as the body adjusts. The source of fuel that the body will turn to is that fat that has been stored in the body.

Fat is much more effective at keeping you full and satisfied and can provide you with a ton of energy in the process. This may take a few days, but by day four or five, you will notice a big difference in the amount of energy that you have when you get on this kind of fast. And as the fat starts to melt off, you will see a big amount of weight come off as well.

Glycogen-bound weight

While your body is used to storing away a lot of your energy in fat reserves throughout the body, it is also going to store some of the energy in your liver and your muscles as glycogen. And just like with the body fat, the reserves of glycogen, along with the water that is bound to them, can end up putting quite a lot of weight on throughout the body.

The amount of extra weight that someone is holding is going to vary between each person, but when it comes to how glycogen is able to affect the weight loss that you get from water fasting, as well as an explanation about how your energy levels behave during fasting, you first need to understand what is going to happen when you go through the first three to five days of the water fast.

The things that will occur include:

- Your body will have a chance to burn through most of the reserves that you have of glycogen.
  Depending on how much glycogen is present in the body, it is possible that you could lose as much as 10 pounds of glycogen bound water weight. This can make the weight loss from this kind of fast look

impressive, but remember that this is water weight, rather than body fat and weight loss.

- After the body has gotten rid of all its reserves of glycogen, realize that you may feel a bit weak and dizzy. Glycogen is the main way that the body is able to store energy, and when these reserves are wiped out, you are going to be a little low on energy.
- You won't be able to get to the higher levels of fat burning as long as there are some glycogen stores in the body that it can rely on for energy. It often takes 3 to 5 days to really make this happen, but if you go on a one-day fast, you should then move into the fat burning process.

Sodium-bound weight

When it comes to the American diet, you will notice that sodium is a really common mineral in the diet, unless you are on a diet that is low sodium. Just like glycogen, sodium is able to bind to water pretty well. This means that the more sodium you take into your diet, the more water weight you have to deal with in the process.

Since you won't be getting any sodium into your diet when you are on a water fast, the body gets a chance to throw away all of the extra of this nutrient that you are carrying around. If you switch from a standard modern diet that is high in sodium to a water fast, you can easily drop up to four pounds of sodium-bound water weight.

This amount is going to vary based on how high your diet was in sodium, to begin with. Also, it will also work to make your final water fasting results look amazing on paper, but again, remember that this is not showing that you are burning off any body fat in the process.

Digested food

If you go on any kind of diet when you first get started, even on a diet where you are allowed to eat some solid foods, you will always have a few pounds of food that have been partially digested and is hanging around your digestive tract. However, when you go on a water fast and you stop eating solid foods completely during that time, you will find that the colon and the digestive tract are able to move on through and empty out. Of course, this is going to take at least two or three days before you see the results.

In fact, it is common for some people to go through a colon cleanse while they are on or before their water fast. This would help to speed this process up a bit and could get rid of more toxins than before. Whether you do a colon cleanse or not, it is still possible to drop a few pounds because some of the food that you have digested is going to leave during the water fast, and you won't take in any food to replace it.

Depending on how much you ate before the fast and how long you go through with the fast, you could lose up to 7 pounds of non-fat weight just because the colon is able to empty itself out a bit more than usual. This can help to make the results of your weight loss if you go on the fast for a week seems even more impressive.

How much weight am I likely to lose on a water fast

Now, the amount of weight that you are likely to lose will depend on a number of factors. To start, if you are male or female, you will lose weight at a different speed. The speed of your metabolism can have something to do with it as well. Even the amount of weight you have to lose from the start, the duration of your water fast, and more.

Let's take a look at some examples of how all of this can work for you by doing a few calculations on how much weight you could reasonably lose when you are on this kind of fast. You will need the table below in order to help you do this calculation or any calculation that you want to complete with these fasts.

Water Fast duration (days)	Weight loss - women (%)	Weight loss - men (%)
1	0.5	0.8
2	1.4	1.8
3	2	2.6
4	2.8	3.4
5	3.5	4.1
6	4.1	4.8
7	4.5	5.2
8	5	5.6
9	5.5	6.2
10	5.9	6.6
11	6.1	6.9
12	6.5	7.3
13	6.8	7.6
14	7.1	7.9
15	7.4	8.3
16	7.5	8.5
17	7.9	8.8
18	8.1	9.2
19	8.4	9.5
20	8.6	9.9
21	8.9	10.2

Our first example is going to be for women. We will say that you are a 150-pound woman who wants to go on a water fast that will last for seven days. You would estimate out the amount of weight that you would lose during this time by taking the value that is in the second column for the seven-day water fast in the table, and then you multiply it by your current weight. So, the formula you would use in order to get an estimate for your weight loss on a seven-day water fast would include:

150 lbs. * 4.5/100 = 6.75

For our second example, we are going to look at the numbers that men may get for this same kind of formula. This time, we are going to look at how much weight a man who weighs 180 pounds will lose if they go on a water fast for fourteen days. You would be able to estimate the amount of weight loss that comes from the water fast by taking the value that is in the third column and lining it up with the amount that is there for the fourteen-day fast. Then multiply this by the current weight and divide by 100.

180 lbs. * 7.9/100 = 14.2 lbs.

As you can see, these are basic formulas that you are able to use in order to figure out how much weight you are likely to lose when you go on a water fast. Each person is going to lose a different amount of weight depending on how much weight they have to lose, how long they are on the fast, and more. Be aware that these numbers are just estimates. Some people may lose more weight, and some may lose less weight depending on the situation at hand.

4

Anti-aging

ANOTHER BENEFIT that you can get when you go on a water fast, or just add more water into your daily life, is to prevent aging throughout all parts of the body. No one wants to deal with aging. There are countless aging creams, other aging tools, and vitamins out there that are meant to help you to look and feel younger. Many of these are going to be quite expensive, and the jury is out on whether they actually do the work that they promise.

You will find that instead of spending all that money and time on creams and other tools that don't provide you with the benefits that you want, you can choose to enjoy more water and get the benefits instead. In fact, going on a water fast and making sure that you drink enough water on a day-to-day basis, you will be able to slow down the aging effects on the body. Let's take a look at how water can be the answer that we are looking for when it comes to preventing aging and looking and feeling our best.

The aging process

We get old because our bodies are not able to properly dispose of all the wastes and toxins that are inside. These wastes and toxins end up accumulating inside the body and can cause a lot of problems. In order for the body to function in a normal way and even to maintain body temperature, we need to burn off nutrients within the cells. The main ingredients in all foods, no matter what kinds we consume, are going to be some combination of fats, proteins, and carbs. To break it down even further, they are going to be nothing but the combination of four main elements including oxygen, hydrogen, nitrogen, and carbon.

After these nutrients are burned up through the cells using them, they will then turn into some of the organic acids. Some examples of these organic acids include ammonia, fatty acids, lactic acids, uric acids, and carbonic acids. Fats are acidic even before they get started with the process of oxidation. To prove this, the word in Chinese for oxygen has been written with two characters of "sahn-so" which literally translates into an acid root.

These acidic wastes and the various toxins are going to be disposed of out of the bodies in some liquid form, either as urine or as sweat when we perspire. This happens after the acids have been dissolved into the blood. Every element that is inside of our body was moved around and placed in its current location by the blood. And it can move to some-where new by first getting dissolved back into the blood and then carried out. If anyone was able to lose ten pounds through dietary means, it is possible to say that most of this weight came out through the urine.

Unfortunately, our current environments and our lifestyles make it very hard to get rid of the various acidic wastes that are there. We end up building too many of these acids in the body, and then the body isn't able to get rid of them to start with. Due to consuming too much food, working too much, indulging in things too much, staying up too late, not sleeping and resting enough, not getting enough exercise, not taking in enough water, being in pollution, and smoking, it is really hard to eliminate the wastes out of the body in a timely manner. We have to accumulate all of these waste products that are left over somewhere inside the body. This is the process of getting old and of aging.

To make the situation worse, mixed in with these organic acids that we talked about above, there are going to be some inorganic acid minerals. These may include things such as sulfur, phosphor, and chlorine. These acids are going to come with some of the foods that we eat that are considered the most acidic, such as root crops, grains, and meats. We don't spend enough of our time eating alkaline or anti-aging foods, like vegetables and fruits, to counteract these. The minerals that are found in these alkaline foods, like potas-sium, sodium, magnesium, and calcium, can really help to reduce the issue that comes with the acids that are taking over. When we miss out on those foods, the acids are allowed to build up, without any help with reducing them until you increase your consumption of fruits and vegetables.

Although the amounts of inorganic minerals are going to be small compared to the acid wastes that the body is going to naturally produce, they can do a lot to contribute to your health. One thing to note is that even if you don't eat any kind of acidic food if you consume proteins and carbs, the body is going to produce more of these acidic wastes than the alkaline minerals are able to counteract.

Now, the body is meant to be more alkaline than anything else. We are born with a pH that is 7.44, which means that we are highly alkaline. Although as we get older, the pH is going to drop down to 7.35 or below. The amount that this drops down is going to vary from person to person based on their lifestyle choices.

The blood pH that we are discussing here is going to be known as the artery blood pH. The difference of just 0.009 in pH level may seem like a small thing, but since this is going to be logarithmic, the amount means that the change is 1.23 times less alkaline than at birth.

In addition, the hydroxyl ion is going to be an oxygen donor, while the hydrogen ion is going to take the oxygen away. In other words, it is common for younger people to have up to 23 percent more of these oxygen donors in their blood compared to older people. Is it any wonder that younger people are more youthful and energetic compared to those who are older?

Another thing to consider is uric acid. This acid is going to be pretty much insoluble in ether, alcohol, and water, but it will be soluble in solutions of alkaline salts. What this means is that uric acid can become soluble when placed in alkaline water.

If you have dealt with issues of gout and arthritis, you know what a pain lot of uric acid can be. These two diseases are going to be caused when uric acid makes its way between the joints. And it won't be dissolved and reduced because the older person (who is more likely to suffer from these issues), doesn't have enough alkalinity in their blood. Drinking acid-free, alkaline water is slowly going to elevate your pH levels, and it could help gout and arthritis to disappear on its own.

As we continue to live with this poor waste disposal system for longer periods of time, it is likely that you will find some areas of your body are accumulating more acids compared to others. And these can end up clogging up the capillary vessels around those kinds of acidic areas. What this does is cause some of the organs in the body to function in a manner that is more sluggish.

We may start to feel tired and run down for no good reason, and some common disease in adults, such as allergies, asthma, diabetes, arthritis, and high blood pressure will start to set in. And because of our age, we simply accept these as they are and assume that they are just a part of getting old, rather than trying to do anything about them.

If the buildup of this acid ends up getting too extreme, it can start to destroy some of the healthy cells that are found around them. In order to keep the cells healthy, they need to maintain a pH level that is slightly alkaline. Some cells will make some changes to their formula in order to make it through the acidic environment. If they do make these changes and are successful, this means that you have the beginnings of cancer.

Cancerous cells are acidic, while cells that are healthy in the body are alkaline. Even if the cancerous tumors are completely removed surgically, as long as the conditions remain acidic, the chances are that new tumors are going to develop in the same area.

Now, the exact place where these leftover waste products are accumulated can vary for each person. However, the areas of the body where these wastes start to accumulate first can sometimes help you to determine what adult disease you are most likely to develop first. Within one family, the storage places are likely to be very similar. This may be able to explain why some adult diseases have a strong hereditary link.

Since the accumulation of waste products inside the body is one of the main reasons for aging, helping the body learn how to get rid of some of the old wastes inside can be the first step in the process of anti-aging, no matter what age you are when you get started.

This kind of process can take you two steps. The first step to see anti-aging effects is to develop a disposal system that is good. The second step is to make sure that all of the old wastes have been pulled out from all of their hiding spots.

Creating a good disposal system

The first thing that we are going to take a look at here is developing a good disposal system to make sure those toxins and wastes are able to leave the body. Since, as we mentioned a bit before, the waste disposal of the body is done through perspiration and urine in a liquid form, it is so critical that we drink lots of water, which is where the water fast can come into play.

When you decide to go on any kind of diet plan, whether it is a fast or not, your doctor and anyone on the diet plan is going to tell you to drink at least 8 glasses of water each day. The reason that they do this is that they know that the disposal of all that waste and those toxins is done through the urine, but they aren't going to tell you what kind of water that you should drink.

Remember, we discussed how all waste products in the body are going to be acidic. As a result, the best water that you should consume, especially when you are trying to prevent aging with the help of a water fast, is acid-free, alkaline water. Drinking four glasses of this kind of water that is alkaline will be more effective of using 8 glasses of regular, filtered, or bottled water. There are some devices that you can use from home, which are known as water ionizers, that are able to split the acid and alkaline minerals through electrical means in your regular tap water.

A quality water ionizer can take in the regular tap water, which is going to have both alkaline and acidic minerals in it. In fact, the typical value of the pH that you will find in your tap water is 7. This system will then release water that has a pH value of 9 or higher with all of the alkaline minerals from the original tap water. At the same time, it is going to release the water that is acidic, which means that the water has a value for pH that is five or lower into the original tap water.

Since this alkaline water has twice as many of these kinds of minerals as the original water that came from the tap and now it has no acidic minerals, it is going to be at least twice as potent as just drinking the water straight from the tap.

Inside our bodies, it is going to be able to just go through and neutralize the acidic elements before helping to discharge them safely from the body. What this can mean for you is that by simply drinking eight glasses of regular tap water, you are going to leech out both the acidic wastes and some of the valuable alkaline materials that need to be there, including the ever-important potassium. This is why many doctors are going to take the time to test out your blood when you are going on a serious diet program. With this alkaline water, there is no need to worry that you are going to lose potassium out of your system, which can help you fight to age even more.

With our modern world and modern lifestyle, you will find that it is hard to dispose of the waste properly. When we don't work out, when we eat the wrong foods, and when we deal with stress, lack of sleep, and pollution, it is easier to build up the acids that are in our lives, rather than being able to reduce them at all.

Water fast can be one of the best ways to ensure that you will see the results you are looking for with anti-aging. It can help you to get started on a healthier lifestyle, which is sometimes all we need to create a good disposal system and help out bodies to stay healthier and happier overall. Try it out. It is best to go on one of these kinds of fasts for about a week to ten days, but even one to three days is a good start and it can help you reduce the effects of aging in no time.

How a water fast can help

As we have spent some time talking about through this guidebook, the free radicals, wastes, and toxins that build up in your body are going to cause a lot of harmful diseases in the body. And one place that they are really going to cause some trouble is in the process of aging. Those who maintain a more acidic environment in their bodies will find that those wastes need to be stored somewhere, and that place is often going to cause a lot of aging effects.

Now, aging can show up in many different forms. For example, it is not uncommon for aging to not only show up in your skin, forming wrinkles, and fine lines throughout the face and other parts of the body. It can also cause issues when it comes to some diseases that are considered "adult" or "aging" diseases. Issues like arthritis and gout are seen as diseases that occur as you get older, but you don't have to let these come and take over your life. If you are careful with your diet and learn how to use water to get rid of some of the acidity in your body, you are going to see some amazing results.

First, one way that your water fast is going to be able to help prevent aging is through preventing or treating the wrinkles and other fine lines that show up in your skin and face. Many people will purchase a lot of pills and skincare products in order to get rid of these lines, but you may be able to use a water fast in order to help you lose those wrinkles and look younger than ever.

In addition to some of the different reasons we will talk about in a minute, drinking plenty of water can help you to provide more hydration to the body. Many times, even when we aren't on a fast, we don't give the body the amount of hydration and water that it needs to maintain its health. This can result in the body feeling worn out, dried out, and more. Taking in the amount of water that you need can hydrate the body and ensures that you are able to get the number of nutrients to the skin that you are looking for.

In addition, you will find that drinking lots of water can help you to prevent aging even more because it will get rid of the toxins and the acids that are in the body. We discussed this a bit before, but the body is not meant to be as acidic as we usually let it. In fact, the body is supposed to be a little bit alkaline in order to stay healthy and help with the normal waste removal that happens inside the body.

When we allow the body to become acidic, this is when the aging starts to come into play. The longer that the body remains acidic, the worse the problems can be. You will find that the acid in the body will build up, won't allow any healing of the cells, and can cause a lot of damage in the long run. You will find that as the acid keeps building up and doesn't get a chance to leave the body, the issue can get worse. This is where wrinkles and fine lines, gout, arthritis, and other conditions that are considered a part of aging will start to become prominent.

This doesn't mean that you have to let it happen. It is perfectly possible for you to get rid of these symptoms of aging, you just need to be able to find a way to reduce the acid in the body and get it to more of an alkaline setting. There are a number of ways that you are able to do this, but one of the most effective and least costly methods is to go on a water fast.

Now, it is possible for you to just increase the amount of water that you consume in your daily diet, work on elimi-nating the amount of acid containing foods that you enjoy in your diet, and you can help reduce the amount of acid in the body. In spite of that, this method is going to take longer to accomplish. The fastest method that can help with this is to go on a water fast.

With a water fast, you make sure that you aren't taking in any foods or drinks that are acidic. This is going to make it so much easier for you to reduce the acid because it can naturally cut itself out to start with. Then, if you are able to find distilled and alkaline water, you can do an even better job at reducing some of the effects of aging.

If you want to get the benefits of this, and you are worried that aging is one of the main reasons that you want to go on this kind of fast, then it may be best to go with a water fast. And you will need to go on the fast for a bit longer than normal. While a shorter water fast is easy to work with when it comes to practicing this type of fast, or when you just want to restart yourself, you will find that the best way to reduce the amount of acidity in the body, is when you need to go on a fast that lasts about seven to ten days instead.

This will give the body some time to get plenty of alkalinity into it and reduce the acidity that is in there as well. When the fast is done, you must make sure that you keep limiting the amount of acidic food that you consume, and you must make sure that you continue to drink plenty of distilled and alkaline water in the process. Without doing this, you will end up causing the acidity to come back up again, and you will run into trouble with aging again.

Going on a water fast can be a very effective method that you can use in order to help you prevent the aging process. Instead of just letting the body get old and dealing with the different diseases that come with it, you can use a water fast and some of the benefits that come with it in order to make the body healthier and to prevent aging. You will find that with proper alkaline water fast, you can reduce the amount of acidity in the body, in order to increase your overall health.

Healing Your Own Body

FASTING IS A COMPLETELY natural healing therapy that has been used by a lot of different societies and cultures for thousands of years. It has been used as a tool to help aid, treat, and sometimes cure many maladies. Even though it is not used as commonly today as in the past, the process of fasting, including water fast, is still going to create some of the same healing as effective today as they did in the past.

And while modern medicine is often trying to alleviate the outer symptoms when it comes to the different health conditions that we deal with, fasting is going to affect the healing from the inside out. Getting to the actual source of the condition, helping to burn out the inferior cells in the body, and building up new cells and tissues that are healthier, is all a part of going on water health.

You will be amazed at the things that the body is capable of doing. In fact, if you give the body the right space and time and you stop feeding it the wrong foods and being stressed out too much, the body is able to start its own perfect healing. Fasting allows you to use that opportunity so that it is able to heal in the perfect way.

So, what are some of the different things that a water fast can do for your body? We have already spent a bit of time talking about the different ways that fasting is able to help you out. Some of the other benefits that you can choose to work with when it comes to using fasting to heal your body include:

- Can help you to heal a bunch of major and minor health conditions that you have been dealing with
- Can be a great way to help you start your own weight loss and can even help you to keep it off
- Cleans your body of all the metabolic toxins and wastes that are present in the body.
- Can improve your skin tone and health, will make you look younger than ever before
- Can help to stimulate new growth of cells in the body, which can make you feel younger
- Strengthens the immune system and the body's own natural defenses, which can help you get sick less often
- Improves your hormonal balance and your glandular health
- Can increase the amount of mental clarity that you deal with on a regular basis
- You will find that water fast, even one that is short-

term can help you have a better mood, and can help you enjoy a more positive outlook

- People who go through a water fast will give you more enthusiasm and energy.
- Will even help to enhance your spiritual connection

There are a lot of other ways that a water fast is able to help your body and keep it in the best health possible. In fact, this is the single best way to ensure that the body is able to avoid a lot of bad diseases and illnesses because these dead cells that cause inflammation and other problems are now going to be eliminated out of the body. When this happens, it allows for more room for the body to do the job that it should and can promote natural healing throughout the body.

Water fasting is a type of fasting that will restrict everything that enters your body except for water. It has become a popular method in recent years in order to help individuals to lose weight quickly. Studies have shown that going on a water fast could have a bunch of health benefits, as long as it is done in the proper way. It could lower the risk of many chronic diseases, and it could stimulate the process of autophagy or the process that will help the body break down and then recycle old parts of the cells.

With that being said, the human studies that have been done concerning water fasting are pretty limited. And it is easy for many people to do the water fast in the wrong manner, which could lead to health risks in some individuals. In this section, we are going to take a look at some of the benefits that come with water fasting and why some people claim it is the best way to lose weight.

Of course, there are a lot of other benefits that come with a water fast, and as you will see, it is going to be one of the most effective ways for your body to start healing itself. Let's take a look at some of these different benefits and determine why water fast may be the best option for you.

It can promote autophagy

While we explored autophagy in a previous chapter, a water fast can help to promote the process of autophagy. Autophagy is the process where the old cells and other parts of the body are broken down and then recycled. This helps new cells to form and can keep the body working much better than before. There are actually several studies that find that proper autophagy throughout the body could help protect against various diseases such as cancer, Alzheimer's disease, and even heart disease.

For example, autophagy has the power to prevent damaged parts of the cells from sticking around and accumulating in the body. This issue can be a big risk factor when it comes to many types of cancers. When autophagy occurs properly, it could be a method that will help prevent cancerous cells from growing in the first place.

Can lower your blood pressure

Research has shown that going on a longer fast that is supervised by a medical professional could really help people who are dealing with high blood pressure get those numbers down. In one of these studies, 68 people, all of whom had borderline high blood pressure, fasted for about 14 days with medical supervision.

When the fast was complete, about 82 percent of those participants saw that their blood pressure was able to fall to healthier levels (120/80 mmHg). Additionally, the average drop in blood pressure of that group was 20 mmHg for systolic (which is the upper value) and 7 mmHg for diastolic (which is the lower value), which is a huge amount for the time that passed.

Yet this isn't the only study that has been done to determine how effective a water fast can be on high blood pressure. In a second study, 174 participants, all of whom had high blood pressure, when on a water fast for ten to eleven days. When the fast was done, about 90 percent of the people in the study were able to achieve a reading that was lower than 140/90 mmHg, which is the limit that is used to diagnose someone with high blood pressure. In addition, the average fall in the participants for the systolic blood pressure ended up being 73 mmHg overall.

The only problem here is that there aren't really any human studies that have been done in order to see how a short water fast, one that is between 24 and 72 hours, would affect blood pressure. All of them so far have been between 10 to 14 days long, but if you are dealing with high blood pressure and would like to work on getting the numbers down, it may be worth your time to consider longer water fast to help.

There is one study that has been done that looks favorable when it comes to water fasting and how well your hypertension will behave. In one clinical trial looking at water fasting and hypertension, 174 people with hypertension were pre-fasted for 2 to 3 days. In this study, they were allowed to eat a few fruits and vegetables. After that time, they then went on a water fast that lasted for 10 to 11 days. And finally, they followed a six to seven-day post-fast, where they would eat low sodium and low-fat vegan diet.

In the initial blood pressure before the study, the participants were in excess of 140/90 mm Hg. By the end of the trial, more than 90 percent of these participants were able to get way below this number. In fact, the higher the initial blood pressure at the start of the study, the more that it was able to drop during this kind of fast. And the average amount of drop in this study ended up being 37.13. Those who were in stage three hypertension, which meant that they had blood pressure readings that were over 180.11, saw an average reduction of 60/17.

Everyone who went on the study had been taking medication for their blood pressure, and when they were done with the fast, they were able to go off that medication.

Fasting has been shown to work well for hypertension in a number of clinical trials, including the ones that we have talked about in this section. In fact, fasting is now believed to be one of the best methods to use in order to lower high blood pressure and normalize cardiovascular function. In addition, the blood pressure tended to stay low in all of those who used fasting to protect their hearts, even after the fasting was done.

Since high blood pressure is a huge issue for many Americans, it can really cause issues with your health and your heart, and how well it is able to work. Being able to lower the high blood pressure and get it down to normal levels can do wonders for your overall health. When you go on a fast, you can effectively get your blood pressure down to normal levels, protect your heart, and feel better overall.

Can help improve the leptin and insulin sensitivity in the body

Insulin and leptin are both important when it comes to the hormones that will affect the metabolism of the body. Insulin is going to be there to help the body store up the nutrients it needs from the bloodstream. And leptin will be there to help your body feel full when you are done eating.

There has been research done that shows how water fasting can actually help you have a higher sensitivity to insulin and leptin. What this means is that these hormones are going to be more effective in the body because the body will respond to them better than ever before.

For example, when you are more sensitive to insulin, it means that the body will become more efficient at reducing the blood sugars that show up in the bloodstream. On the other hand, having a higher sensitivity to leptin could help you to process the hunger signals more efficiently and can lower the risk of obesity.

For those who are worried about weighing too much and who are looking to lose some more weight, the increase in leptin sensitivity can be a great thing. It helps you to have a better idea of when you feel full and can keep you on track with your own eating habits. When it comes to insulin, having a higher sensitivity to insulin can help prevent and even reverse the harmful effects of diabetes in the body.

Can help you lower your own personal risk of many chronic diseases

There has been some evidence in the past that shows how going on a water fast could help lower the risk of chronic diseases throughout the body. Some of the chronic diseases that may fit into this category include heart disease, cancer, and diabetes.

In one of the studies that took a look at the effect of water fast on these chronic diseases, 30 healthy adults went on one of these water fasts for a 24-hour period. After the fast was done, these individuals had significantly lower blood levels of triglycerides and cholesterol, two of the biggest risk factors when it comes to heart diseases.

In addition, there have been several animal studies that have found that being on a water fast could protect the heart from the damage that free radicals in the body could cause. These free radicals are basically molecules that are unstable and tend to damage the different parts of the cell. They are sometimes the primary cause of chronic diseases.

In other animal studies, it was found that water fasting had the power to suppress the genes that help the cancer cells to grow. In some cases, when it was used properly and under the supervision of a doctor or medical staff, good water fast could help to improve the effects of chemotherapy.

Can help the body clean itself out

As we talked about a bit with the process of autophagy, your body can use the time that you are on a water fast in order to clean itself out and promote self-healing. The current modern lifestyle makes it very hard for the body to function properly. We take in a lot of free radicals, eat the wrong foods, and worry about things too much, and this can make it hard for the body to function in the proper manner.

When we keep going with this kind of lifestyle, it becomes hard for the body to clean itself out. Dead and damaged cells are a normal part of the body. Things break down or get damaged all the time, but because of the unhealthy lifestyle that many of us are living with today, the body isn't able to eliminate those dead and damaged cells.

Instead, they get stuck inside the body, and they cause more damage. They move around and cause some damage when it comes to the rest of the body. And they get in the way of the body making new cells that can help you heal. This just keeps building upon itself and can make the situation worse many times.

When you go on a water fast, you are giving the body some time to clean itself out, and that promotes self-healing. The body has the tools that it needs in order to do that, but sometimes it needs the time and a little break in order to get it done. Focusing on just drinking water, even for one or two days, can be the trick that you need to see results.

Now, we spent some time taking a look at the different studies that show how effective water fast can be to cleaning out the body and making you as healthy as possible, but the human studies are still pretty limited when it comes to the total impact of water fasting. It is necessary for more research to be done before this becomes a regular thing for most people, and it is often recommended that you talk about this kind of fasting with your doctor, especially if you have some major health concerns.

Water fast and helping with seizures

There have been some preliminary studies done that show how going on a water fast could be beneficial for those who are dealing with chronic epilepsy. This can include reducing the length of the seizures, the number, and the severity. Fasting, even water fast, can be especially effective when it comes to helping alleviate or cure childhood epilepsy.

This could be due to the fact that the body is changing the

primary fuel source and relying more on fat, similar to what is done in the ketogenic diet. Even a shorter fast can do some wonders for helping solve this issue. For those who are dealing with epilepsy and the conditions that come with it, it may be time to talk to your doctor and see if going on a water fast could help you to deal with the problem.

Help solve pancreatitis

In a trial that was done in 1998, 88 patients who were dealing with acute pancreatitis. These individuals who had this issue found that fasting was better than any other medical intervention that was used during that time. In fact, neither cimetidine or nasogastric suction would produce the same kind of benefits that come from fasting. And regardless of the etiology of the disease, fasting was able to help out quite a bit.

Arthritis

Many different types of arthritis were able to see relief when it came to going on a water fast. In fact, there have been a number of studies that show how fasting can be effective for dealing with rheumatoid arthritis and osteoarthritis. Fasting is able to induce a number of anti-inflammatory actions in the body, and researchers found decreased ESR, pain, stiffness, and the need for medication.

Arthritis is a big issue that a lot of people will have when they start to age. There are a number of reasons that these types of arthritis can start to flare up and cause issues. The biggest reason is inflammation from the free radicals and the dead cells get in the way, and make it hard for the body to repair itself. Getting rid of those old cells and the free radicals through a detox like a water fast can make a big difference.

In addition, the same thing is going to happen with a variety of autoimmune diseases, and for the same reason. Some autoimmune diseases such as lupus, acute glomerulonephritis, chronic urticaria, and rosacea can all see a great response when it comes to fasting. If you are suffering from any form of arthritis or some common autoimmune diseases, it may be worth your time to try out a water fast to see how that can help you feel better.

Improves your immunity

There are so many reasons why you want to make sure that your immunity is nice and strong. It helps you to feel better. It ensures that you aren't going to get sick as often. You are able to miss fewer days at work, spend more time with your friends and family, and spend more time enjoying the things that are the most important.

With the traditional American diet, it is pretty much impossible to keep the body healthy. You are causing inflammation throughout the body with all the dead and damaged cells that are causing a lot of harm in the body, and the immunity is trying to fight off that issue. And you aren't providing the body with the nutrients that it needs to stay healthy, which suppresses the immunity even more.

You will find that your poor immune function will improve when you go on a water fast. Studies have found that when you are on a fast, you can see an increased amount of macrophage activity, an increased immunity in the cells, a decrease in complement factors, increase in the levels of immunoglobin, and more. All of these come together to help you get a better immune system than ever before and can make you feel amazing.

If you are dealing with a lot of issues that come from your immunity or you feel that you are always sick, then it may be time to consider going on a water fast. Even going on one for just a few days, you will be able to see some amazing effects to your immune system. If you are able to add it into your routine and you start to do a water fast on a regular basis, you will find that your immune will get stronger than ever before.

Water and heart disease

You may be surprised to find out, but water is one of the best tools when it comes to fighting against the harmful effects of heart disease. Researchers from Loma Linda University in California confirmed that this is true when they spent some time checking the water intake of 20,000 participants aged between 38 and 100 as a possible risk factor for fatal coronary artery disease. Again, in a 2002 study, it was found that water was a strong protector against heart disease, regardless of gender.

To be sure, these studies can only provide us with an indication of whether water is effective at helping with heart disease, and they will never be outright proof of cause and effect. What is interesting with these kinds of studies though is that the researchers from them found that elevated viscosity or blood thickness, the volume of red blood cells, and the fibrinogen, which is the protein involved in helping blood clot, number of individuals who drank less than two glasses of water each day was common compared to those who drank five glasses or more.

When these factors are elevated, even when they are at the high end of the normal range, they can lead to a higher risk of coronary heart disease. These are going to make your blood thicker, which is something that can be found between diabetic and heart patients. In addition, these elevated values were found years before this kind of heart conditions started showing.

Viscosity can be a really big deal here. It is important, but often it is a big risk factor when it comes to cardiovascular disease. The thicker the blood is, the slower it is going to be able to flow through the circulatory system. In the process, this thick blood can cause a lot of issues such as inflammation, cardiac trouble, plaque, and clots. Your heart has to work harder to push that thicker blood through your veins. You will also find that this thicker blood will contain a lot of excess insulin and glucose, bacteria, and toxins, along with some other harmful substances that bring about inflammation and can damage the blood vessels if it is left untreated. A good way to think about this is that your blood is healthy when it seems more like wine, rather than ketchup.

Being dehydrated is the most common cause of this higher viscosity. However, the research says that you should just flood the blood non-stop with water, but it does help if you learn how to drink enough water so that you don't become dehydrated. When you are doing this, it becomes easier to avoid issues with the viscosity, and it can do some wonders for making your blood and heart stronger than ever before.

With that said, a water fast is able to help protect your heart in so many ways. As long as you make sure that you are drinking enough and not getting dehydrated, you may be able to protect your heart. Water fast helps to lower blood pressure, clear out the toxins, and can do so much to make the heart strong. In addition, going on a fast for a week or more can help train you in how much water you should be drinking every day to keep yourself as healthy as possible. When you bring that into your daily life, you will find that it is easier than ever to protect your heart. And it all comes from drinking enough water.

Improved cell recycling

Autophagy is the body's normal and natural process for recycling any components that are dysfunctional or unnecessary. The body is able to do this on its own, but sometimes we need to give it a break from free radicals and an unhealthy lifestyle, including eating, in order to allow the body some time to get started with this process.

Water fasting can be a good way to force the system into a state of autophagy. With the caloric intake severely reduced, your body is going to become more selective in which cells it is going to protect overall. What this means is that a water fast is able to encourage your body to heal naturally, and the body will start to actively destroy and then recycle some of the damaged tissues that often get in the way. As a result, the body may get some relief from several serious health conditions.

There is a lot of anecdotal evidence that comes from individuals who claim that water fasting is able to help them overcome a lot of disorders that had taken over their lives. And many of these claims have now been backed up by research. In addition, animal studies have shown that going on an alternate day fast, that could include water fasting, was able to reduce the incidence of cancer and metabolic syndrome.

The dangers and risks of water fasting

Now that we have spent some time talking about all of the benefits of going on a water fast, and all of the cool things that can come with this kind of fasting, it is important to note that it isn't always the best idea to go on with this. Individuals who are healthy, who don't go on the fast for too long, and who are careful that they follow the fasting rules the right way, will do just fine with this fasting method. Those who are not that healthy, who spend too long on the fast and don't listen to their own bodies, and who decide that they know best and don't follow the rules, are going to run into some trouble.

Although water fasting can have some benefits, there are also a few health risks that come with it as well.

Some of the risks and dangers that can show up when you work with water fasting if you aren't careful may include:

You may lose weight, but it could be the wrong kind

Since going on a water fast is going to restrict how many calories you get to eat, you are going to be able to lose a ton of weight very quickly. In fact, there is research that shows how you could lose up to 2 pounds each day of a one to two-day water fast if you do it the proper way. Depending on the amount of weight that you are trying to lose, you may be able to lose even more for the few days you are on the fast.

However, you may not be losing the kind of weight that you want. When most people go on a diet and exercise plan to lose weight, they are focusing on reducing the amount of fat that they trim off the body. While you may be able to lose a bit of fat when you get started, a lot of the weight that you will lose during this time, especially during some of the longer fasts, would include water, carbs, and muscle mass instead.

It is possible to become dehydrated on a water fast

Although this may sound strange since you are going on a fast that includes only water, it is possible for this kind of fast to make you feel dehydrated. This is because about 20 to 30 percent of the water that you take in each day will come from the different foods that you eat. If you spend your fast only drinking the same amount of water that you did to start with, but you don't eat any foods, then it is possible for you to not take in the amount of water that your body needs to keep going.

It is important for you to increase the amount of water that you are consuming each day. A few extra cups can make a big difference in the risk that you have for dehydration. You should also be on the lookout for any signs of dehydration that may start to creep in. Always look out for low levels of productivity, lower blood pressure, constipation, headaches, nausea, and dizziness.

The risk of orthostatic hypotension

While some people do decide to go on a water fast in order to reduce their high blood pressure, it is sometimes possible that those who go on a water fast will suffer from orthostatic hypertension. What this means is that there is a sudden big drop in blood pressure that happens when you stand up quickly. This drop in blood pressure can make you feel light-headed, dizzy, and can put you at an increased risk of fainting.

If you find that you go on a fast and then suffer from this kind of disorder, then it is important to avoid operating any heavy machinery or even driving when you are on this kind of fast. The risk of fainting and dizziness can end up causing an accident if you are not careful. If you find that the situation gets too bad, it is time to get off the water fast.

If you have a medical condition, the water fast can make it worse

Although most water fasts are going to be pretty short, unless you do one under medical supervision, there are several conditions that seem to get aggravated when you go on a water fast. People who suffer from the following medical conditions should be careful about going on a water fast, and should discuss doing this kind of fast from their doctor before they even get started:

- Gout - Water fasting has the ability to increase the production of uric acid. This is a big risk factor for gout attacks. If you have issues with gout already, then a water fast may not be the right option for you.
- Diabetes - Fasting has the power to increase the risk of adverse side effects in those who are suffering from type 1 and type 2 diabetes.
- Chronic kidney disease - In some cases, water fasting is able to cause more damage in the kidneys for individuals who are suffering from chronic kidney disease.
- Eating disorders - There is also a bit of evidence that shows how fasting of any kind, whether it is water fasting or another type, could encourage a variety of

eating disorders, including bulimia, especially for teenagers.

- Heartburn - It is possible that fasting could trigger some common issues like heartburn. This is because the body is going to keep on making lots of stomach acid, but now that you are on a fast, there isn't any food for the acid to digest, therefore you may suffer from heartburn.

Although water fasting can have a lot of great health benefits, there are some dangers and risks that you need to be aware of. For example, if you are not careful with the kind of water fast you go through, it is possible that this kind of fasting could make you more prone to blood pressure changes, dehydration, and muscle loss, along with some other serious health conditions. It is always best to talk to your doctor before you get started with this kind of fasting.

How to Go on a Water Fast

NOW THAT WE have spent some time in this guidebook talking about a water fast and some of the amazing benefits that can come with even a short-term fast, it is now time to delve a bit deeper and look at some of the specifics of going on a water fast. Yes, even something that seems as simple as a water fast does have some rules to follow to make it more effective and to ensure that you still maintain your health. For example, long-term water fasts, such as over ten days, shouldn't be done often, if at all, and when they are, they should be done under the supervision of a medical professional to ensure you are staying healthy and not in any danger.

However, there is more to it than that. Knowing how much water to drink, how long you can go on the fast, and more can ensure that you really do get the most out of this kind of fasting. Let's take a look at some of the things that you can consider when it comes to starting your very own water fast.

The steps to getting started on a water fast

When you go on a water fast, it is very important that you are careful with the kind of water that you drink. This is the only thing that you will consume during this kind of fast, so you want to make sure that the type you take in is fresh, clean, and of the highest quality. Since you aren't consuming anything else for this time, any contaminants in your water will be magnified inside the body. It is often recommended that you go with distilled water and nothing else during this kind of fast.

Some people who go on a water fast will choose to drink filtered water because that is the easiest for them. If you have a good filtration system in place for this, then that is fine to choose that option, but you will find that the distillation process is going to go further than filtration and can remove more harmful chemicals and organisms. And if your filtration system isn't the best, you may still have a lot of contaminants in the water. It is best to go with the distilled water if possible.

The next step and often one of the most important steps is to arrange your schedule during this fast. If you can, take some time off of work for the duration of the cleanse, or schedule it during a time when you are going to be home anyway. This way, you won't be tempted by all of the food that may end up in the break room, and if you feel a little tired and light-headed, it is easy to get some more water and lie down. Most of these fasts are only going to be for a few days so fitting them in during a weekend, or just taking off a few days usually is pretty easy to do.

From there, you need to choose how long you would like to do the water fast for. You can technically do the fast for up to a month, but for most people, especially those who have never done a fast before, this is going to be way too long, and it is not recommended that you start with that long. The most common length for the fast includes one, three, five, seven, or ten days. Start out small with this one so that you can get used to the idea and can give your body time to adjust. One to three days of fasting in this manner can be effective as well and is a great way to get started.

If you plan to go on a fast that will last for longer than five days, or you are fasting to help you gain control over some serious conditions, you may want to consider getting some supervision for your water fast. Many people do this for at least the first few times that they are on a fast because it offered them an environment that is more controlled, a team of professionals who will watch them and help them if something goes wrong with their health condition, and other people who are going on the fast as well and who can provide emotional support.

For those who have medical conditions, it may be a good idea to visit a fasting clinic before you start. This kind of clinic can do some tests to find out the best type of fast for you, it can help you to monitor how your health is doing during a fast, and can ease you back into solid foods if you happen to go on a fast that is too long.

Now, before we get started with being on one of these water fasts, there are a number of precautions that you should take. Keep in mind that most people who choose to go on a water fast are just fine and they receive all of the benefits and more than we have listed in this guidebook, but it is still important to take these precautions to ensure that your body stays strong and healthy, and to ensure that you get the benefits that you are looking for when you go on a water fast.

First, make sure that you do not go on a water fast, any other fast, or restrictive diet when you are pregnant or lactating. A child who is developing is going to be way too sensitive to nutritional deficiencies and when you go on this fast for more than a day, they will notice and may suffer in the process as well. Wait until the baby is born and after you are done breastfeeding before you decide to go on one of these water fasts.

In addition, anyone who is suffering from type 1 diabetes may benefit from going on a different type of detox plan. You are limiting yourself too much on one of these kinds of diet plans, and it could be hard on a body that is dealing with diabetes at the same time. If you think that you would still benefit from this kind of fast while you are dealing with type 1 diabetes, talk to your doctor. They may be able to discuss the benefits and the things to watch out for and may recommend that you do a supervised fast if they find that it would be beneficial for your needs.

And finally, make sure that you are not underweight when you get started with fasting. Most of those who see the best with water fasting are those who are at least 20 pounds overweight. If you are less overweight than this, or you are a healthy weight and just want to get some of the other health benefits, then you will need to be careful about the way that you fast. You can still try it out and see, but make sure that your first fast is a bit shorter than others.

What should I do before the water fast

It is important to prepare yourself before you even get started on one of these water fasts. This is a fantastic way to help you see some results with fasting, and can ensure that you aren't going to run into any issues while you are doing the fast.

The first thing that you should do in order to get started with a water fast is talk to your doctor about it. This is a great way to help you take a look at some of your health conditions and determine if the water fast is actually something that is a good idea for you. Most people will be just fine when they go on these fasts, but there are some conditions, such as pregnancy, breastfeeding, and type 1 diabetes to name a few that can get worse when you go on one of these fasts. Talking to your doctor ahead of time can make it easier for you to get the results that you want without worrying about your health at the same time.

Next, you need to decide how long you would like to be on the fast. These fasts usually go between one, three, five, seven, and ten days. Longer fasts should really be used under the supervision of your doctor and not on your own. Picking out one of these other time limits is best when you want to do this all on your own to get the benefits.

If you are worried about how the water fast will go or this is your first time on any good diet plan, then it may be best to go with a one or three-day fast. This does give you some benefits, especially if you plan to stick with it and do one on a regular basis, and it allows you to have a good chance of getting used to the whole process.

In addition, you may find that going on a longer fast is better for you. Many of the benefits that you are looking for when it comes to water fasting is to go on one that is about seven days long. If you plan to go on a fast that is this long, you should plan things out and make sure that you are able to get as much rest and relaxation as possible during this time.

And finally, you need to prepare your diet ahead of time. Don't go on an incredibly intense diet plan before the fast because you need to have a few nutrients built up inside the body before you are able to get started. Although you can plan things out a bit. For example, if you are looking to go on a water fast in order to lose weight and burn fat, you may consider going on the ketogenic diet a few weeks before you start the water fast. This will ensure that you are already in the fat burning mode before you start with the fast, and this can make it more effective. In addition to losing the other weight types that we talked about above, being on the ketogenic diet before starting a water fast can ensure that you will reach the fat burning state and see even better results.

What should I expect when I go on my first water fast

When you go on a fast, it is important to remember that this is more of a time for resting, not for a lot of exertion. This is why we recommended that you try to take some time off, or at least plan the fast during the weekend or another time when you could take things a little bit easier.

Many people go on a water fast because they want to lose a lot of weight, and they think that by eating nothing and running themselves super hard, they will be able to get a lot of extra benefits and lose even more weight. Yet you will find that this is hard on the body, and not something that you should do. Since you are limiting the calories that you eat during this time, the body is going to be lower on the nutrients that it needs to stay healthy. Hard workouts need carbs and other nutrients to keep going. And just by breathing and being alive, your body will use up the extra stored nutrients pretty quickly.

Now, if you take it easy, you won't see that much of a difference in how you feel other than your energy levels may be a bit lower than before. This is not the time for you to go out and try to do the heavy lifting, a marathon, or any other hard and intense workout regimen. The body simply doesn't have the nutrients that it needs to do that work.

When you are on the fast, you need to just rest and relax. Don't even think about going to the gym; you can live without it for a few days. You may find that the body is tired and wants to sleep more than usual. And it is just fine to let yourself sleep a bit more while you are on this fast. This is the time when you need to listen to your body, so take naps and rest during the day as much as you need. Don't be alarmed by this because it is just a part of the process. Relax and embrace the results that you will get.

During this time, you need to make sure that you drink enough water each day. This ensures that the body is able to do what it needs to and that you won't get dehydrated in the process. Depending on your body and how busy you are, you need about 2 to 3 quarts of water for each day that you are on the fast, but make sure you don't drink it all out at once. Space this amount over the day so that you are hydrated properly and you can also increase your satiety, so you don't feel as hungry during the fast.

Now, be aware that for the first few days of the fast, things may be a little bit tough. You may notice some symptoms that are uncomfortable, such as disorientation, headaches, irritability, and hunger. This is also why you should stay at home during the fast. It allows you time to relax so you don't feel overwhelmed and you can deal with those side effects at the same time.

The good news here is that the body is resilient and if you go on the fast for more than one or two days, it is going to adapt pretty quickly. You will notice that you feel a lot better when you enter the third and the fourth day. In some cases, some participants in the water fast will report feeling some euphoria when they get to this point and they find the last few days easier to handle.

If you notice that the symptoms aren't getting better or they get too hard to handle and you start to feel sick, it may be time to cut out the water fast a little bit early. This fast is meant to help you feel better and to improve your health, not make you feel sick. Yes, it does take a little bit of time to adjust to the water fast and to go a few days without eating food, but it isn't supposed to make you feel sick. Listen to your body and make sure that you are handling the fast in the proper way so you can get the most benefits.

Tips and tricks for your water fast

Going on a water fast is not meant to be a difficult process to go with. You simply cut out all the foods and drinks that you consume outside of water. This will help you to feel your best and get all of the benefits that come with this kind of fast. Some of the tips that you can follow in order to get the most out of your water fast includes:

- Read - You will quickly find that a book can be your best friend when you work on a fast. When you are fasting, you need to be able to rest your body, while also finding ways to keep your mind busy and occupied so you don't give in and eat during the fast.

This means that your fast is a good time to catch up on all of that reading you haven't had time for. It is low in energy, but really entertaining; therefore you can keep busy.

- Set realistic goals - When you get started with your water fast, make sure that you are realistic about the goals that you set. Think about why you are doing this kind of cleanse. To help a particular health issue? Are you trying to do it to lose weight? Set simple, clear, and achievable goals that match with what you want to get out of the fast.

- Meditation - Meditation can be nice here because it reinforces willpower and will promote a healthy connection between your mind and your body. Many people find that when they spend time meditating, they are able to control their cravings and do a better job at strengthening their resolve. Others report that hunger will distract them and they have trouble with meditating. You have to figure out what works best for you.

After the fast

At this point, you have probably been on the fast for at least a few days. No matter how long you go on the fast for, you need to make sure that you end that fast in a safe and effective matter. As you end your water fast, resist the urge to go in and overindulge, especially if the fast was a long one.

With a fast that only lasts for one or two days, this won't be as big of an issue. However, if you go on a fast that is a week or more, you need to be extra careful about what you do as you end your fasting, especially when you are in the first few days. While it is normal to dream about eating anything in your path after going without any food, your rebooted digestive system is just not going to be able to handle that. Your stomach has been emptied for some time now, and you may find that eating too much food, or foods that are too rich, can cause you severe discomfort, and even some serious complications.

It is much better for you to break your fast in a slow manner. Start by just drinking juice and Detox water, then move on to broths, and then slowly add in solid foods. This should be done over the course of a day if you went on a fast that was shorter, such as ones that are only a few days long. If you were on a fast that lasted between three to seven days, you must wait 24 hours before you introduce the solid foods back into your diet.

And if you went on a fast that was over seven days, you may want to wait between 36 and 48 hours before you introduce the solid foods back in. Remember that this fast can be a process that takes several days, just listen to your body and make sure that you don't take on more than you are able to handle.

Fasting is a fantastic way for you to go through and reset your system, while also bringing in a ton of health benefits, but remember that it is not a way to cheat an unhealthy lifestyle. You can't expect to eat as much as you want and overindulge all of the time, and then just go on a water fast on occasion to cancel out that damage. Instead, water fasting needs to be done as part of a healthy lifestyle overall.

This means that you need to make sure that you pick out healthy lifestyle choices when you are done with your water fast. Consider other lifestyle choices that you should make when it comes to being healthy such as fresh fruits and vegetables, getting lots of rest, exercising on a regular basis, learning how to manage stress, and avoiding environmental toxins. You should definitely use your water fast as a start or an opportunity to abandon bad habits and add in some new healthy habits to your routine.

How long should I fast for

It is best to determine how long you should be on the fast for ahead of time. This helps you to have some resolve when it happens and can help you to prepare in case you feel tired. Most people find that it helps to take some time off work or to do the fast on their days off so they can relax and feel better during that time.

The amount of time you take to go on the fast is going to vary based on a number of factors. If this is your first fast, going on a shorter one is going to be the best, unless you have some severe medical conditions that you are hoping to solve with this kind of fast. A one to three days fast can be a great way to experience what this fasting is about, and can still give you some results.

After you have had some time to set up the fast and get used to the way that fasting works on you, it may be time to extend the fast. Many of the studies that have been done on the benefits of water fasting were done over a time period of seven to ten days. This can be your goal to get a lot of great benefits, but for someone who is just starting out, it may seem a little bit daunting. Getting started slowly and building up is a better way to go.

No matter the length you decide to choose for your fast, decide on this amount ahead of time and make some adjustments so you know what is going to happen and can prepare. This type of fasting does take out some energy, and you may feel tired and worn out in the beginning. Don't worry, this is normal and the body will adjust, but this is why we recommend that you take it easy as you get used to the fasting process.

What if something goes wrong

For the vast majority of people who go on a water fast, nothing is going to go wrong when they are on a fast. In fact, after the first few days on the fast, you will feel so much better. You will feel lighter as some of the weight and the toxins start to fade off. You will have more energy as the body starts to rely on your fat stores for energy, instead of glucose and the body parts are able to start feeling better than ever before.

However, in some cases, the body may not react the way that you would expect. Some people don't react as well to these fasts as others, and they may have to change things up a bit. This is where you must learn how to listen to your body before you get started on the fast. If you start feeling too weak and sick on the water fast, it may be time to cut it short. You don't want to ruin your health or cause other issues along the way.

If you feel that the water fast has gone incredibly wrong, then it is time to talk to your doctor. They will be able to help you manage the fast in the proper manner. They can also help make sure that you don't get dehydrated and that any medical conditions that are affected by the fast are still kept under control.

There are many great things that you will get when it comes to working with a water fast. You can put the body into the process of autophagy, and that process alone encourages the body to heal itself and results in a ton of fantastic health benefits. No matter what goals you are trying to reach with your health, a water fast will be able to help you get there.

Conclusion

Thank for making it through to the end of *Water Fasting: Autophagy, Weight Loss, Anti-aging, and Healing Your Own Body Fast for Beginners*. Let's hope it was informative and able to provide you with all of the tools you need to achieve your goals in whatever they may be.

The next step is to decide when the right time it is to go on the water fast for yourself. This guidebook spent time looking at what water fasting is all about, the benefits of autophagy, and more and has provided you with the research that you needed to understand just how powerful this kind of fasting can be. Even going on the fast for just a few days can make a world of difference in your weight loss and even how you feel overall.

There are a lot of different types of diets out there, and even different types of fasts that you can choose to go on, but water fast is often seen as one of the most effective methods.

It eliminates all types of food for a certain period of time and the only thing that the person can have is water. It is important that during this time you take in extra water than usual since you are missing out on some of the water you naturally get from food. Outside of that, many people find that a water fast can be extremely effective for them.

The length of the fast is going to vary based on the individual and their needs with this kind of fast. Many people do one-day fasts to reset their bodies and prepare them for a new diet plan and lifestyle plan. Some do alternate day fasting where they will do this kind of water fast every other day, or at least a few days a week, in order to help them lose weight and be healthier.

Then there are longer fasts as well. There have been studies that show how well this kind of fasting can be even at 14 days, though these types of fasts should be done with the help and supervision of medical professionals to make sure that your body stays healthy. No matter what type of water fast you go on, you will see tremendous results and will wonder why you didn't try this out sooner.

This guidebook went into details about going on a water fast and how effective it can be for your overall health. It can help to fight off aging, can help you to lose weight, and can do wonders for how well the body is able to clean itself and heal itself, effectively cutting out a lot of the harmful diseases that have taken over and caused a lot of issues.

While water fasting isn't for everyone, including those with severe medical issues and those who are pregnant or nursing, it can be incredibly effective when it comes to a healthy individual who is trying to help their body go through some of its normal processes. If you have been looking for a way to lose weight, get rid of some illnesses and diseases easier, and just get yourself in the best health possible, make sure to check out this guidebook and learn everything that you need to know to get started with your own water fast.

Finally, if you found this book useful in any way, a review on Amazon is always appreciated!